Contemporary Concepts in the Diagnosis of Oral and Dental Disease

Guest Editor

IRA B. LAMSTER, DDS, MMSc

DENTAL CLINICS OF NORTH AMERICA

www.dental.theclinics.com

January 2011 • Volume 55 • Number 1

SAUNDERS an imprint of ELSEVIER, Inc.

W.B. SAUNDERS COMPANY
A Division of Elsevier Inc.

1600 John F. Kennedy Boulevard • Suite 1800 • Philadelphia, Pennsylvania 19103-2899

http://www.dental.theclinics.com

DENTAL CLINICS OF NORTH AMERICA Volume 55, Number 1
January 2011 ISSN 0011-8532, ISBN-978-1-4557-0434-7

Editor: Donald Mumford; D.Mumford@elsevier.com

Dental Clinics of North America (ISSN 0011-8532) is published quarterly by Elsevier Inc., 360 Park Avenue South, New York, NY 10010-1710. Months of issue are January, April, July, and October. Business and Editorial Offices: 1600 John F. Kennedy Boulevard, Suite 1800, Philadelphia, PA 19103-2899. Periodicals postage paid at New York, NY and additional mailing offices. Subscription prices are $240.00 per year (domestic individuals), $420.00 per year (domestic institutions), $113.00 per year (domestic students/residents), $287.00 per year (Canadian individuals), $529.00 per year (Canadian institutions), $347.00 per year (international individuals), $529.00 per year (international institutions), and $170.00 per year (international and Canadian students/residents). International air speed delivery is included in all *Clinics* subscription prices. All prices are subject to change without notice. **POSTMASTER:** Send address changes to *Dental Clinics of North America*, Elsevier Health Sciences Division, Subscription Customer Service, 3251 Riverport Lane, Maryland Heights, MO 63043. **Customer Service (orders, claims, online, change of address): Elsevier Health Sciences Division, Subscription Customer Service, 3251 Riverport Lane, Maryland Heights, MO 63043. Tel: 1-800-654-2452 (U.S. and Canada). Fax: 314-447-8029. E-mail: journalscustomerservice-usa@elsevier.com (for print support); journalsonlinesupport-usa@elsevier.com (for online support).**

Reprints. For copies of 100 or more, of articles in this publication, please contact the Commercial Reprints Department, Elsevier Inc., 360 Park Avenue South, New York, NY 10010-1710. Tel.: 212-633-3812; Fax: 212-462-1935; E-mail: reprints@elsevier.com.

The *Dental Clinics of North America* is covered in *MEDLINE/PubMed (Index Medicus), Current Contents/Clinical Medicine, ISI/BIOMED* and *Clinahl.*

Printed and bound by CPI Group (UK) Ltd, Croydon, CR0 4YY
Transferred to Digital Print 2011

Contributors

GUEST EDITOR

IRA B. LAMSTER, DDS, MMSc
Dean and Professor of Dental Medicine, College of Dental Medicine, Columbia University, New York, New York

AUTHORS

TARA AGHALOO, DDS, MD, PhD
Associate Professor, Oral and Maxillofacial Surgery, University of California Los Angeles School of Dentistry, Los Angeles, California

CHRISTOS ANGELOPOULOS, DDS, MS
Associate Professor and Director, Oral and Maxillofacial Radiology, Columbia University, College of Dental Medicine, New York, New York

RENY DE LEEUW, DDS, PhD
Associate Professor; Chief, Division of Orofacial Pain, College of Dentistry, University of Kentucky, Lexington, Kentucky

ELLEN EISENBERG, DMD
Professor and Chair, Section of Oral and Maxillofacial Pathology; Director, UConn Oral Pathology Biopsy Service, University of Connecticut Health Center, Farmington, Connecticut

DEEPTHIMAN GOWDA, MD, MPH
Course Director, Foundations of Clinical Medicine, College of Physicians and Surgeons, Columbia University, Presbyterian Hospital, New York, New York

CATHERINE H.L. HONG, BDS, MS
Department of Oral Medicine, Carolinas Medical Center, Charlotte, North Carolina

IRA B. LAMSTER, DDS, MMSc
Dean and Professor of Dental Medicine, College of Dental Medicine, Columbia University, New York, New York

PETER B. LOCKHART, DDS
Chair, Department of Oral Medicine, Carolinas Medical Center, Charlotte, North Carolina

DANIEL MALAMUD, PhD
Professor of Basic Sciences, Department of Basic Sciences, New York University College of Dentistry; Professor of Medicine, Department of Infectious Diseases, New York University School of Medicine, New York, New York

LOUIS MANDEL, DDS
Director Salivary Gland Center; Associate Dean and Clinical Professor (Oral and Maxillofacial Surgery), Columbia University College of Dental Medicine, New York, New York

EASWAR NATARAJAN, BDS, DMSc
Assistant Professor, Section of Oral and Maxillofacial Pathology, University
of Connecticut Health Center, Farmington, Connecticut

JEFFREY P. OKESON, DMD
Professor and Chair, Department of Oral Health Science; Director, Orofacial Pain
Program, College of Dentistry, University of Kentucky, Lexington, Kentucky

JAMES J. SCIUBBA, DMD, PhD
The Milton J. Dance Head and Neck Center, The Greater Baltimore Medical Center,
Baltimore, Maryland

KENNETH J. SPOLNIK, DDS, MSD
Clinical Professor and Chair, Department of Endodontics, Indiana University School
of Dentistry, Indianapolis, Indiana

MYCHEL MACAPAGAL VAIL, DDS
Clinical Assistant Professor, Department of Endodontics, Indiana University School
of Dentistry, Indianapolis, Indiana

DENISE E. VAN DIERMEN, MD
Clinic for Medical-Dental Interaction, Academic Center for Dentistry Amsterdam (ACTA),
Amsterdam, The Netherlands

DANA L. WOLF, DMD, MS
Assistant Professor of Clinical Dental Medicine, Section of Oral and Diagnostic Sciences,
Division of Periodontics, Columbia University College of Dental Medicine, New York,
New York

ANDREA FERREIRA ZANDONA, DDS, PhD
Associate Professor, Department of Preventive and Community Dentistry, Indiana
University School of Dentistry, Indianapolis, Indiana

DOMENICK T. ZERO, DDS, MS
Professor and Chair, Department of Preventive and Community Dentistry; Director,
Oral Health Research Institute, Associate Dean for Research, Indiana University School
of Dentistry, Indianapolis, Indiana

Contents

> When first case examples presents to a dentist, a patient may have a specific complaint, be in need of routine evaluation, or arrive on referral from another health care provider. In all cases, proper diagnosis of existing problems is the essential first step in provision of appropriate oral health care. The clinician's approach to diagnosis and the need to arrive at the appropriate diagnosis are daily challenges in dental practice. This article discusses the prescriptive and descriptive theories of diagnostic reasoning using 4 case examples.

> Although all dentists are taught about the importance of oral health to general health and that systemic disease can manifest in the oral cavity, the 4-year dental school curriculum does not allow time to gain competency in these relationships. Nevertheless, all dentists must have skills in taking a medical history and an appreciation of oral findings that might have a systemic origin. This article focuses on the identification of abnormal signs and symptoms in the oral cavity and the determination of those that have a systemic origin. It is imperative that clinicians are mindful of the possible oral-systemic associations, because these could potentially have a huge impact on patient care.

> This article reviews the diagnostic process, from the first clinically evident stages of the caries process to development of pulpal pathosis. The caries diagnostic process includes 4 interconnected components–staging caries lesion severity, assessing caries lesion activity, and risk assessments at the patient and tooth surface level - which modify treatment decisions for the patient. Pulpal pathosis is diagnosed as reversible pulpitis, irreversible pulpitis (asymptomatic), irreversible pulpitis (symptomatic), and pulp necrosis. Periapical disease is diagnosed as symptomatic apical periodontitis, asymptomatic apical periodontitis, acute apical abscess, and chronic apical abscess. Ultimately, the goal of any diagnosis should be to achieve better treatment decisions and health outcomes for the patient.

> Periodontitis is an inflammatory disease of bacterial origin that results in the progressive destruction of the tissues that support the teeth,

specifically the gingiva, periodontal ligament, and alveolar bone. The diagnosis of periodontal disease currently relies almost exclusively on clinical parameters and traditional dental radiography. In this article, the authors review current diagnostic techniques and present new approaches and technologies that are being developed to improve assessment of this common condition.

This article addresses several issues in the approach to diagnosis of oral cancer. The term oral cancer is clarified. Key aspects of the biologic basis of development of oral cancer and the known risk factors associated with the disease are summarized. The clinical presentation of oral cancers and precancerous lesions and their histopathologic correlates is discussed. The importance of conventional tissue biopsy as the prevailing gold standard for diagnosis is emphasized. Other current technologies available for detecting and diagnosing oral cancer and premalignant lesions are acknowledged, and their respective strengths and weaknesses are discussed.

This article discusses the classic autoimmune diseases: pemphigus vulgaris, mucosal pemphigoid, and oral lichen planus. These are generally considered of autoimmune origin or, at a minimum, immune system mediated. Cause, diagnosis, and treatment are discussed. As management of these diseases progresses, continued advances in molecular pathogenesis will allow insight into which strategies can be employed in interfering with the complex cascade of events leading to mucosal impairment and clinical morbidity.

There are many types of pain conditions that are felt in the orofacial structures. Most of the conditions treated by the dentist are associated with the teeth, periodontal structures, and associated mucosal tissues. This article focuses on the differential diagnosis of other common pain conditions the dentist will likely face, such as temporomandibular disorders, neuropathic pain disorders, and common headaches; and the clinical presentation of each. Controlling or reducing pain can be accomplished by controlling perpetuating factors such as parafunctional habits and by some simple behavioral modifications. Finally, this article offers some simple treatment considerations.

Salivary gland abnormalities and salivary dysfunction are important orofacial disorders. Patients with such problems are usually seen in the dental office for evaluation and therapy, and the dental practitioner is required to make a diagnosis and institute care. Therefore, it is necessary for the dentist to be knowledgeable regarding the more common pathologic entities that involve the salivary apparatus, and also be familiar with the diagnostic and therapeutic tools that are available. Successful diagnosis is dependent on the organized integration of the information derived from past history, clinical examination, salivary volume study, imaging, serology, and histopathologic examination. This article discusses the most common disorders seen in the Salivary Gland Center and indicates the current approaches to diagnosis. Improvement in diagnostic skills will avoid serious complications and lead to specific and effective therapy.

Imaging Technology in Implant Diagnosis

Christos Angelopoulos and Tara Aghaloo

Dental implantology based on osseointegration is among the most significant advances in dental science in the last 50 years. Imaging technology contributes to all stages of implant treatment, from presurgical site evaluation to postoperative assessment of integration, and long-term periodic evaluation of implant status. Various imaging modalities have been used for dental implant assessment in the different stages of implant treatment. These include intraoral radiography (film-based and digital), panoramic radiography, computed tomography, cone-beam computed tomography, and others. Selection of the specific imaging technique should be based on its suitability for providing the diagnostic information required by the implant team at different stages of treatment. This article reviews the applications of different imaging technologies and their diagnostic contribution to presurgical evaluation, treatment planning, and postoperative assessment of dental implants.

Saliva as a Diagnostic Fluid

Daniel Malamud

Salivary diagnostics is a dynamic and emerging field utilizing nanotechnology and molecular diagnostics to aid in the diagnosis of oral and systemic diseases. In this article the author critically reviews the latest advances using oral biomarkers for disease detection. The use of oral fluids is broadening perspectives in clinical diagnosis, disease monitoring, and decision making for patient care. Important elements determining the future possibilities and challenges in this field are also discussed.

RELATED INTEREST

Oral and Maxillofacial Surgery Clinics of North America
February 2010 (Vol. 22, No. 1)
Clinical Innovation and Technology in Craniomaxillofacial Surgery
Bernard J. Costello, DMD, MD, FACS,
Guest Editor

THE CLINICS ARE NOW AVAILABLE ONLINE!

Access your subscription at:
www.theclinics.com

Preface

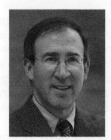

Ira B. Lamster, DDS, MMSc
Guest Editor

Diagnosis is the essential first step in the provision of health care. A patient presents to a health care provider for a routine evaluation or with a specific complaint requiring attention. The provider will review the health history, ask pertinent questions about the history and symptoms, and then examine the patient. This will be followed by the use of other diagnostic procedures and tests, which can include radiographic studies and analysis of biologic fluids and tissue samples. Arriving at the correct diagnosis allows for selection of appropriate treatment, with minimal time delay. Health care providers must continually seek to improve their diagnostic acumen.

Diagnostic procedures in dentistry have relied heavily on clinical measures and standard radiographic assessment of the mineralized tissues (teeth and bone). Today there is a renewed emphasis on diagnosis of oral and dental diseases. In part, this is because oral inflammation may have adverse affects on tissues and organs at distant sites. In that same vein, there has been a focus on analysis of saliva as a diagnostic fluid. Further, new devices and instruments are being introduced for the evaluation of different oral diseases, including oral squamous cell carcinoma and dental caries. This new technology is in the process of being evaluated, and some of these devices will ultimately be incorporated into dental practice once their utility is verified.

This research will focus the dental profession on the importance of arriving at the correct diagnosis, which will mean devoting more time and energy to this first phase of patient care. This volume will contribute to this new emphasis by reviewing current and forward-looking approaches to the diagnosis of oral, dental, and craniofacial diseases and disorders.

A monograph cannot possibly address the diagnosis of all diseases and disorders of the oral cavity and its contiguous structures. Nevertheless, as evidenced by the articles in this issue of *Dental Clinics of North America*, the complete oral health care provider must be familiar with pathology of the teeth, gingiva, oral mucosa, the mandible and maxilla (including the temporomandibular joint), muscles of mastication, and the salivary glands. Further, in the United States and other western countries these disorders occur in a population that is aging, becoming more medically complex, and

Dent Clin N Am 55 (2011) ix–x
doi:10.1016/j.cden.2010.08.011
0011-8532/11/$ – see front matter © 2011 Elsevier Inc. All rights reserved.

dental.theclinics.com

using an ever-expanding number of medications. The comprehensive diagnostic evaluation of patients seen in the dental office depends upon consideration of the patient's health history and health status.

A fundamental issue that influences the relative importance of diagnosis in dental practice is the reliance on a coding system that identifies the treatment that is required, but not the diagnosis of the disease or disorder. In medicine, the International Classification of Disease, Ninth Revision, Clinical Modification (ICD.9.CM) is a coding system used to identify diagnoses, and current procedural terminology (CPT) is used to identify the treatments that are performed. In contrast, dentistry utilizes current dental terminology (CDT) codes to bill for services, but the diagnosis is not routinely supplied.

The use of diagnostic codes, and a focus on diagnosis as the driver of any proposed treatment plan, is more than just a different means to an end. A new emphasis on accuracy and specificity of the diagnostic process will certainly be enhanced with the use of diagnostic codes. In fact, diagnostic codes for oral and dental disorders have been developed (ie, the Systematized Nomenclature of Dentistry, or SNODENT) but this system is not currently in use. Introduction of a diagnostic coding system will better align the dental profession with medicine in regard to the focus on the patient's problems and provide other advantages such as allowing population-based analyses of oral disease trends.

The focus of both our educational system and clinical practice is on procedures that restore lost or damaged tissues. The modern oral health care provider will also need to become equally proficient in the diagnosis of a wide range of diseases and disorders affecting the oral cavity and its contiguous structures. This will require a paradigm shift that must begin with dental education and be continuously emphasized in clinical practice. Further, compensation for the examination and diagnostic phase of oral health care must be increased. This will be a tangible incentive that emphasizes the importance of the diagnostic evaluation. The result of these changes will be improved oral health care outcomes and better alignment of dentistry with the health care system.

Ira B. Lamster, DDS, MMSc
College of Dental Medicine
Columbia University
630 West 168th Street
New York, NY 10032, USA

E-mail address:
ibl1@columbia.edu

The Diagnostic Process

Deepthiman Gowda, MD, MPH[a],*, Ira B. Lamster, DDS, MMSc[b]

KEYWORDS

- Bayes theorem • Diagnostic reasoning • Heuristic thinking

When first presenting to a dentist, a patient may have a specific complaint, be in need of routine evaluation, or arrive on referral from another health care provider. In all cases, proper diagnosis of existing problems is the essential first step in the provision of appropriate oral health care. The clinician's approach to diagnosis and the need to arrive at the appropriate diagnosis are daily challenges in dental practice. This challenge can be daunting given the complex anatomy of the oral cavity and its contiguous structures. Please consider the following case:

CASE 1

A 42-year-old woman was referred by her physician for evaluation of a painful lesion on her tongue. This discomfort was associated with an ulcerated area on the lateral border (**Fig. 1**). The lesion had been present for 6 weeks, and the patient consulted her dentist. As the lesion persisted, the patient began having difficulty eating and also developed hoarseness. The patient reported using an over-the-counter topical medication containing benzocaine to treat the lesion. She was otherwise well and was not using any medications.

Initially, the dentist suspected several possibilities, but the leading diagnoses were primary herpetic gingivostomatitis and an aphthous ulcer. Other possible diagnoses included an autoimmune disorder and infection (syphilis or tuberculosis). The lesion did not have an erythematous base, making herpetic gingivostomatitis less likely. Certain characteristics of the lesion, primarily the persistence and severity of the ulceration, helped in establishing a diagnosis. The voice change, although not diagnostic, was also suggestive of an autoimmune disease that can affect the larynx. Pemphigus vulgaris was suspected, and a biopsy of the lesion was performed.

The results of the biopsy revealed an intraepithelial split. Direct immunofluorescence was positive within the epithelium. The biopsy results were consistent with pemphigus vulgaris, and the patient was ultimately treated with intraoral topical steroids. Close observation for the appearance of other lesions on the skin, and other symptoms suggestive of more advanced disease, was also recommended.

---

[a] College of Physicians and Surgeons, Presbyterian Hospital 17-105, 630 West 168th Street, New York, NY 10032, USA
[b] College of Dental Medicine, Columbia University, 630 West 168th Street, New York, NY 10032, USA
* Corresponding author.
E-mail address: dg381@columbia.edu

Dent Clin N Am 55 (2011) 1–14
doi:10.1016/j.cden.2010.08.002
0011-8532/11/$ – see front matter © 2011 Elsevier Inc. All rights reserved.

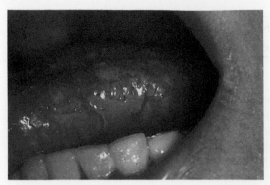

Fig. 1. Lesion on the lateral border of the tongue.

In this case, the dentist considered several conditions that are associated with oral ulcerations, including herpetic gingivostomatitis, aphthous ulceration, and autoimmune disorders such as pemphigus vulgaris. Because the practitioner suspected an autoimmune disorder such as pemphigus vulgaris, a condition with high morbidity if untreated, early biopsy was recommended. Meanwhile, if the practitioner had thought the patient was affected by herpetic gingivostomatitis or aphthous ulceration, the appropriate intervention might have been to provide symptomatic care. Misdiagnosing a case of pemphigus vulgaris as herpetic gingivostomatitis or aphthous ulcer might have resulted in the delay or failure to provide appropriate treatment for a disease associated with significant morbidity. On the other hand, mistaking herpetic gingivostomatitis or aphthous ulcer for pemphigus vulgaris might have led to the unnecessary administration of potentially toxic medications. The clinician in this case relied on a careful history, clinical examination, astute clinical judgment, and an appropriate diagnostic procedure (biopsy) to swiftly and correctly diagnose pemphigus vulgaris.

This case illustrates the profound effect that the diagnostic impression can have on clinical outcomes. Diagnostic reasoning is the process of gathering pertinent clinical data from the history, clinical examination, and other testing; distilling meaning from that information; and then formulating an appropriate diagnostic hypothesis.[1] A great deal has been written about how clinicians solve diagnostic problems. Although diagnostic skill is central to the endeavor of providing quality dental care, dentistry-specific literature on diagnostic reasoning is surprisingly limited. In this article, the authors describe several key concepts regarding diagnostic reasoning and illustrate these ideas with case studies. Understanding these various theories on the diagnostic process helps clinicians become better diagnosticians.

PRESCRIPTIVE THEORIES

Decision making had been a topic of study in cognitive psychology, philosophy, and mathematics for several decades before it became a topic of scholarly interest in clinical care. Within the field of clinical decision making, the initial wave of research was focused on developing rational or prescriptive approaches to diagnostic reasoning. Researchers sought to explore how practitioners can make the best and most rational diagnostic decisions.

Von Neumann and Morgenstern[2] were among the first to publish in the area of decision sciences with their application of expected utility theory. They argued that people's decisions are based on an individual's assessment of the benefits of choices modified by personal preference, the probability of possible outcomes, and the assessment of and avoidance of risk.[3] Decision analysis emerged as an extension of expected utility theory in which multistep decision making is analyzed. In decision analysis, each diagnostic choice is represented as a node or branching point on a decision tree. Each node is associated with risks, benefits, and utilities for each possible decision.[4] Theoretically, given this set of assumptions, the clinician can proceed rationally through the possible diagnostic choices for a specific clinical situation and arrive at the best possible outcome. One application of decision analysis is in the development of diagnostic decision trees. Thus, if available, the dentist encountering the patient with an oral ulceration (case 1) might reason through the diagnostic possibilities and the need for further workup using a decision tree based on a rational assessment of the clinical factors and the utility of the clinical choices.

CASE 2

A 54-year-old man presented to his dentist with a complaint of pain when chewing on the left side. His medical history included a history of stress, which requires occasional use of the anxiolytic alprazolam (Xanax), otherwise being noncontributory. The intraoral examination demonstrated a slight swelling on the buccal mucosa at the midpoint of tooth No. 30. The examination also revealed a maintained dentition, with the posterior teeth restored with amalgam restorations and crowns. There was mild to moderate wear of the cusps of the posterior teeth.

Radiography of the mandibular left posterior sextant revealed that tooth No. 30 was treated endodontically, that a post was present in the distal canal, and a large radiolucency was present in the furcation area (**Fig. 2**A). The radiolucency was not localized to the area of the post and extended beyond the apices of both roots. Radiography also revealed that the endodontic obturation was inadequate for both roots. No obvious fracture was observed.

The differential diagnosis in this case included an inadequate endodontic obturation, a root perforation related to the post, as well as a localized periodontal lesion. Given the patient's history of anxiety and bruxism, a fractured tooth was included in the differential diagnosis.

Before obtaining the radiograph, the clinician thought that there was an intermediate probability of a fractured tooth. Once the radiograph was available, the clinician must consider the likelihood of a fracture. As mentioned, the radiograph did not demonstrate an obvious fracture. How likely is it that the patient has a fractured tooth, given this finding? The application of Bayes theorem, a statistical rule for combining probabilities, can be helpful in appreciating how information from additional testing affects the likelihood of a particular condition.[5]

The following basic formula describes the concept of Bayes theorem:

Pretest odds × likelihood ratio = posttest odds

Most clinicians can appreciate pretest chances of a disease being present, when it is described as a probability. For instance, if the dentist were to estimate the likelihood of a fractured tooth at 60% before obtaining the radiograph, he or she is describing a probability. The pretest probability refers to the clinician's estimation of the chances that the patient has a given problem before an additional test is performed. In this

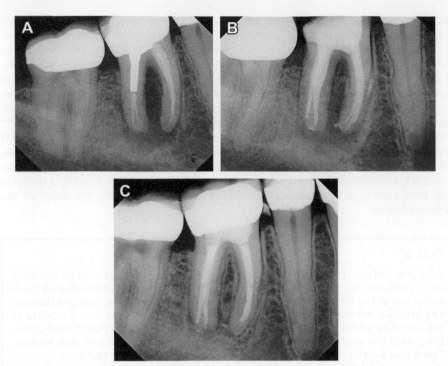

Fig. 2. (*A*) Initial radiographic presentation of tooth No. 30. (*B*) Radiograph taken immediately after retreatment of tooth No. 30. (*C*) Radiograph taken 6 months after endodontic retreatment.

case, that additional test is radiography. The pretest probability is based on several factors, including the prevalence of the condition in the patient's demographic group, the patient's history, clinical examination, and results from previous diagnostic tests. It is to be noted that this estimation is partly subjective and, thus, may vary from dentist to dentist. In this case, because of the history and physical findings, the clinician might have an intermediate suspicion for a fracture before the radiograph is obtained, estimating the pretest probability at 60%. To use Bayes theorem, however, this pretest probability must be converted to pretest odds. A pretest probability of 60% is converted to pretest odds of 1.5 using the following formula:

Odds = probability/1 − probability

The next variable to consider in the Bayes equation is the likelihood ratio. The likelihood ratio reflects how much a positive or negative finding changes the odds of having a given condition. It is a variable that is based on the performance characteristics of the test being used, combining both the sensitivity and specificity values of a test. These test performance characteristics, the sensitivity and specificity, must be available to the clinician in order to use Bayes equation. In this case, the clinician performed a quick literature search to locate a study that reported the sensitivity and specificity of (digital) radiography of detecting a fractured tooth as 86% and 85%, respectively.[6] The sensitivity can be thought of as the proportion of positive test

Table 1 Likelihood ratio of Bayes equation		
	Fractured Tooth Present	**Fractured Tooth Absent**
Radiograph +	A	B
Radiograph −	C	D

Group A, disease and test result positive.
Group B, disease negative but test result positive.
Group C, disease positive but test result negative.
Group D, disease and test result negative.

results among all those patients with the disease. Specificity is the proportion of negative test results among those who do not have the disease. These concepts are represented in **Table 1**.

Sensitivity is calculated as A/A + C and is a measure of how often disease is identified by the test in a total population with the disease. Specificity is calculated as D/B + D, and is a measure of how often the disease-free state is identified amongst those without the disease.

A likelihood ratio is the likelihood that a given test result would be expected in a patient with the disorder of interest compared with the likelihood that the same result would be expected in a patient without the disorder. The sensitivity and specificity of the test of interest can then be combined to calculate the positive and negative likelihood ratios.

The likelihood ratio of a positive test result (LR+) is calculated as

LR+ = sensitivity/1 − specificity

The likelihood ratio of a negative test result (LR−) is calculated as

LR− = 1 − sensitivity/specificity

Using 0.86 and 0.85 as sensitivity and specificity values, respectively, LR+ is 5.7 and LR− is 0.16.

With an intermediate pretest odds of 1.5, a negative test results in a posttest odds of 0.24 (1.5 × 0.16 = 0.24). This posttest odds can then be converted to posttest probability using the following formula:

Posttest probability = posttest odds/1 + posttest odds

This calculation results in a posttest probability of 0.19 or 19% of having a fractured tooth. The absence of an identifiable fracture in the radiograph lowered the probability of fractured tooth from intermediate to low. The test result, in this case, affected the overall clinical impression, and given these findings, the clinician chose to re-treat the tooth endodontically (see **Fig. 2**B). The clinical swelling resolved, and the postoperative radiograph indicated increased density of the bone in the furcation area (see **Fig. 2**C). On the other hand, if the radiograph had shown a fracture, using a LR+ of 5.7, the posttest odds become 8.55, with a resultant posttest probability of 0.90 or 90%. In such a scenario, the practitioner might have chosen to extract the tooth. Thus, in a clinical scenario with an intermediate pretest probability and a diagnostic test with fairly robust test characteristics (high sensitivity and specificity), a test result can have a large effect on the final impression.

It is worth considering the effect of the test result when the pretest probability is very high or very low. If a high pretest probability of 95% or 0.95 is assigned, a positive test result would increase the posttest probability to 0.99 or 99% and a negative test result would lower the probability to 0.75 or 75%. If the pretest probability had been very low, at 0.05 or 5%, a negative test result would reduce the posttest probability to 0.01 or 1% and a positive test result would only increase the probability to 0.22 or 22%.

Two lessons can be gleaned from this scenario. First, the pretest probability, or the patient's history and the clinical examination, modifies the effect of subsequent testing on the final clinical impression. Second, in situations with a very low or very high pretest probability, further testing is not likely to change the clinical impression and may actually lead to false-positive or false-negative conclusions. Even when the sensitivity and specificity of a diagnostic test are fairly high, the test is most valuable in scenarios with intermediate pretest probabilities. Thus, an understanding of bayesian analysis can help the dentist estimate the effect of a diagnostic test on the final clinical impression. In some cases, this understanding might help the clinician decide whether or not to obtain a diagnostic test in the first place.

Limitations of Prescriptive Theories

The use of decision analysis, decision trees, bayesian analysis, and other normative approaches to diagnosis have their limitations, although they are logical and rational tools. For instance, when using bayesian analysis, one must first describe a pretest probability. As mentioned, this estimation is ultimately a clinician's subjective assessment of the likelihood of disease. One practitioner's estimation of the pretest probability of a fractured tooth may differ from another's. The use of bayesian approach is also best suited for a diagnostic test that has a binary set of outcomes, with a positive or negative test result. It becomes problematic when a test result is more ambiguous or measured on a continuous scale (not dichotomous). How should the practitioner apply Bayes theorem when the test result is not conclusively positive or negative; for instance, when the radiograph suggests rather than definitively demonstrating a fracture? Some have argued that arriving at mathematically calculated posttest odds of disease might misleadingly imply a level of precision and scientific certainty to the diagnostic endeavor, which is ultimately subjective. Furthermore, the use of these normative strategies might require the oversimplification of often highly complex clinical scenarios.[7]

The use of decision analysis to understand diagnostic reasoning also has its limitations. Although it seems reasonable to think that clinicians weigh each decision node in a logical fashion, as might be represented by a decision tree, this might not actually reflect how clinicians think in clinical settings. Rather, descriptive literature on diagnostic reasoning reveals that clinicians are often more likely to draw on past experience to make diagnoses and less frequently on carefully constructed logical pathways. Clinicians are sometimes resistant to using decision trees and may consider algorithmic approaches to diagnosis to be overly simplistic.[8] Clinicians might also not think logically about utilities and probabilities. There is evidence that practitioners tend to overvalue risk and possible harm over possible benefits from a given decision.[2] These behaviors are not limited to novice clinicians; even expert clinicians are noted to make decisions that are not in keeping with the logical decisions anticipated by decision analysis theories.[9]

It is possible that these normative diagnostic approaches are not always followed in practice because they have significant costs. For instance, the application of bayesian analysis, evidence-based dentistry, or a rational approach suggested by decision analysis requires time, investment of cognitive effort, and access to real-time information. In practice, the clinician might not have the time, energy, or information needed to formally explore the diagnostic process in the way that is necessary in these approaches. Despite these limitations, later in this article, the use of prescriptive theories of diagnostic reasoning is considered as a solution to some of the pitfalls encountered in typical diagnostic thinking.

DESCRIPTIVE THEORIES

CASE 3

A 51-year-old woman presented with a chief complaint of a swelling on the buccal aspect of the mandibular right first molar (**Fig. 3**A). There was some discomfort, which the patient did not describe as pain. The buccal furcation was probable, suggesting a class II furcation. The posterior teeth were restored with a crown and amalgam restorations.

A periapical radiograph revealed that tooth No. 30 had been treated endodontically, and there was radiolucency in the furcation (see **Fig. 3**B).

The differential diagnosis formulated by a novice clinician included a perforation of the mesial root, root fracture, localized periodontal defect, or neoplastic lesion in the furcation area. An expert would rule out a fracture because of the limited extent of the radiolucency as well as rule out a strictly periodontal problem because the height of the alveolar bone is normal elsewhere in the radiograph and the patient did not demonstrate periodontitis. The chance of a neoplastic process is less. The likely diagnosis was a root perforation on the distal surface of the mesial root.

The patient was treated by excavation of the tooth and removal of the amalgam core. A perforation was identified and treated with mineral trioxide aggregate. Clinically, the fistula resolved, and the furcation observed by radiography improved without periodontal therapy (see **Fig. 3**C, D, and E).

Heuristics and Diagnostic Scripts

Real clinical settings are often hectic and full of distractions. Information may be ambiguous, incomplete, or unavailable, and the clinical scenarios are highly complex. Dentists may be under tremendous time and productivity pressure, requiring diagnostic assessments to be made quickly. How do clinicians reason in these real-world settings? Do they make diagnostic decisions using a conscious, logical, and stepwise process described by decision analysis? Do clinicians explicitly estimate pretest probabilities and consider test characteristics when deciding whether or not to order a diagnostic test? More recent research in diagnostic reasoning has addressed these types of questions and has sought to describe how the diagnostic process actually occurs in clinical practice.

Research suggests that the approach to reasoning differs between experts and nonexperts.[10] As illustrated by case 3, a nonexpert practitioner such as a student explores the history and physical findings in a deliberate and logical fashion. The

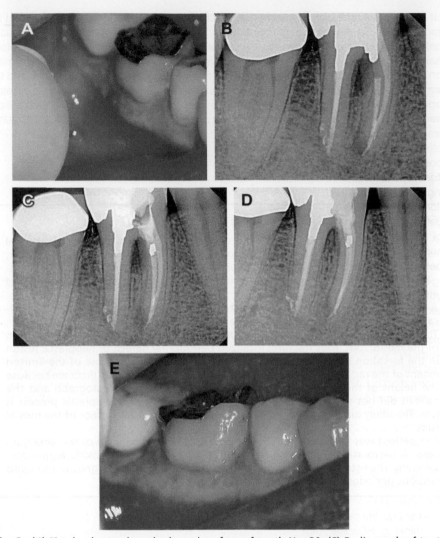

Fig. 3. (*A*) Fistula observed on the buccal surface of tooth No. 30. (*B*) Radiograph of tooth No. 30 at the time of initial presentation. (*C*) Radiograph of tooth No. 30 after identification of the perforation and treatment with mineral trioxide aggregate. (*D*) Radiograph taken 6 months after treatment; radiolucency in the furcation is resolving. (*E*) Resolution of the fistula after treatment of the perforation.

nonexpert then sifts through the information obtained and then tries to make sense of it, consciously constructing a differential diagnosis. In case 3, based on a review of the initial history and clinical examination, the nonexpert clinician might consider a perforation of the mesial root, root fracture, localized periodontal defect, or neoplastic lesion as possible diagnoses. This differential diagnosis affects any further history or examination maneuvers the practitioner wishes to pursue. The practitioner collects all this information and moves to a conclusion based on those findings. This process is iterative, with diagnoses being formulated and affecting information gathering, which then reorders the differential diagnosis. This analytical approach has been described as a hypothetico-deductive reasoning strategy. It is a stepwise, labor intensive, and rigorous process and requires considerable cognitive effort and time.[11]

The expert processes information a bit differently. As soon as the clinician begins to interact with the patient, he or she begins to make conscious and unconscious observations and interpretations. Visual cues as well as verbal and nonverbal information are used in this process. If the clinician has a great deal of experience in a given area, he or she generates a list of hypotheses with little effort. Again, this process occurs both consciously and unconsciously. This list of possibilities then affects the subsequent information obtained by the clinician. In case 3, the seasoned practitioner weighed the available history, examination findings, and radiographic findings and quickly settled on a diagnosis of root perforation on the distal surface of the mesial root. Seasoned practitioners are able to gather information and make clinical assessments very quickly in a vast majority of routine cases and do not have to go through the lengthy hypothesis generation and information gathering in the same stepwise and iterative fashion as the nonexpert practitioner.[12]

This efficiency in diagnostic reasoning observed in expert practitioners is largely possible because of the use of cognitive shortcuts called heuristics. Heuristics represent conscious as well as unconscious recognition of clinical patterns.[1] Some theorists have described the heuristic frameworks used in a clinical context as diagnostic or illness scripts.[13] Each script is formed through clinical experience and learned knowledge and represents a web of information about disease conditions that are associated with typical historical and clinical examination findings. When information is being gathered during a patient encounter, multiple scripts are activated in the mind of the clinician, and the clinician then searches for those scripts that fit the scenario being experienced. This process, called script processing, involves the activation and consideration of several possible diagnostic scripts simultaneously; again, this can be both a conscious and unconscious process. These scripts are narrowed down as more information is gathered through the history, examination, and other testing modalities.[14] The use of this heuristic approach allows the practitioner to quickly assess the case without having to rely as much on the formal hypothetico-deductive reasoning process used by the nonexpert clinician.

Most practitioners use a mix of both heuristic thinking as well as more formal analytical thinking. However, as a practitioner gains experience and more diagnostic scripts are formed, heuristics is likely to play a larger role in the assessment of routine cases.[12] Because of lack of experience and paucity of diagnostic scripts, the nonexpert clinician does not use heuristics as extensively as the seasoned practitioner. Researchers have found that with time, expert practitioners develop more refined illness scripts rather than an enhanced ability to reason.[15]

Some researchers have argued that the ability to form and use heuristics might have been evolutionarily advantageous to early humans.[16] To survive, early humans likely needed to quickly assess and act in fast-moving and perilous situations. Processing and interpreting sensory phenomena using heuristics formed from prior experience and teaching might have allowed these humans to act with speed and effectiveness. Theorists have considered the use of heuristics in diagnostic reasoning as an application of the same cognitive tool to allow the practitioner to function swiftly in a complex and fast-moving clinical environment.[17] However, one can imagine that the use of heuristics can introduce its own set of problems. The following case can be considered.

CASE 4

A 50-year-old overweight woman with no significant prior medical or dental history presented to her dentist with a complaint of bleeding gums and bad breath. She reported that she visited the dentist only periodically, usually when she experienced pain. She stated that she believed she was in good health and did not report using any medications. In the review of symptoms she reported mild fatigue. The patient reported that her father died of a heart attack at the age of 63 years and her mother was alive and taking medication for diabetes mellitus.

The oral examination revealed moderate to severe periodontitis (**Fig. 4**). Ten teeth (Nos. 1, 2, 3, 7, 14, 15, 16, 17, 30, and 31) were missing and not replaced. Several amalgam restorations were present. The gingiva demonstrated moderate to severe inflammation, being most pronounced in the papillae. Periodontal abscesses and moderate plaque accumulations were present. Probing depths ranged from 2 to 10 mm, with generally greater depth associated with the posterior teeth. The remaining molar teeth also demonstrated furcation involvements.

The dentist diagnosed moderately severe periodontitis and began treatment with oral hygiene instruction, scaling, and root planning. The oral hygiene improved, but tissue inflammation remained. The patient then underwent surgical periodontal treatment in the maxillary right quadrant. The healing response was fair, with persistence of inflammation of the gingiva in both the areas treated with periodontal surgery and elsewhere in the mouth. A second periodontal surgery was performed (maxillary left quadrant) with a similar postoperative course. The patient was not seen again for a few months. When she returned to the office she reported that she had been hospitalized for fatigue and dehydration and was found to have had diabetes mellitus (random blood glucose measurement of 355 mg/dL and an glycated hemoglobin [Hb] A_{1c} level of 12.4 % at admission) that had been previously undiagnosed. Since then, her weight was reduced and she was taking oral medications for diabetes mellitus (metformin and glipizide, twice daily). The HbA_{1c} level has decreased to 7.2%. The examination revealed that oral hygiene was improved, and tissue inflammation was reduced when compared with the initial presentation. Periodontal therapy was began again and successfully completed.

So what went wrong in this case? The relationship between periodontitis and the undiagnosed diabetes remained undiscovered. In this situation, heuristic thinking might have led the practitioner astray. The same cognitive shortcuts that led to a quick and correct diagnosis in case 3 may have led to the wrong conclusion in this case. The initial impression was that the patient was afflicted by chronic periodontitis, a condition seen daily in dental practice. This was a reasonable consideration given the high prevalence of the condition and the clinical findings of inflammation and increased probing depth. In most cases, the dentist would have been correct. Indeed, heuristic reasoning used by the experienced practitioner leads to the correct diagnosis most of the time. As the case evolved, however, new developments did not fit neatly with the initial diagnosis. Why was there no improvement with initial treatment and then with surgical treatment? Could the history of fatigue have been important? How about the family history of diabetes? Should these findings have broadened the differential diagnosis? Despite these factors that might have challenged the initial diagnosis, the dentist in this case remained fixed on a diagnosis of chronic periodontitis.

Unchecked heuristic thinking can lead to cognitive biases and diagnostic errors.[18] This case demonstrates 2 common cognitive biases that can be related to heuristic thinking: premature closure and anchoring. In premature closure, the clinician reaches

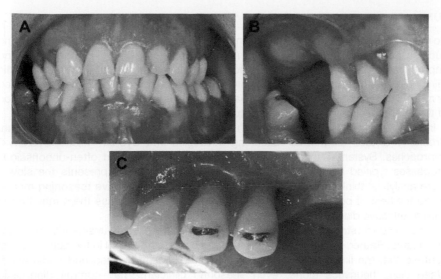

Fig. 4. Initial clinical presentation. (*A*) Anterior view. (*B*) Buccal aspect of the right side. (*C*) Palatal view of the maxillary right lateral incisor, cuspid, and first and second bicuspid teeth.

a conclusion early in the workup of the case, even before all the appropriate information is obtained.[19] This condition is in contrast to the practice of keeping an open mind about the final diagnosis until all the pertinent information is gathered. This case may also illustrate a bias called anchoring that involves a persistent commitment to a diagnosis even though subsequent data contradict that diagnosis.[19] The patient did not improve with the initial treatment and demonstrated persistent inflammation despite improved oral hygiene. Yet, despite this evidence that might have challenged the initial hypothesis, the clinical impression did not change. Both these types of cognitive biases can be a consequence of heuristic thinking and are often found together, as seen in this case.

Unfortunately, the results of unchecked heuristic diagnostic thinking are cognitive errors, which then may result in delayed and missed diagnoses, delays in care, and possibly prolonged suffering. There has been a considerable amount of literature written in the past decade about medical errors and brought to the forefront of national health priorities in large part by the Institute of Medicine report *To Err is Human: Building a Safer Health Care System*.[20] Although this report was mainly focused on medications and systems errors, diagnostic errors are increasingly recognized as an important subset of medical errors. Indeed, diagnostic errors may result in higher rates of morbidity than other types of errors.[21] Although there are several causes of diagnostic errors, such as ineffective information systems, poor communication, and unavailable diagnostic tools, cognitive errors on the part of the clinician are also included.[22]

Heuristic tools might have been effective in navigating the simple systems encountered by early humans but they may not be sufficient as the sole tool for tackling the complex problems encountered in the modern clinical environment. This case implies that the same cognitive tools that allow seasoned clinicians to quickly assess a clinical scenario may in some situations predispose clinicians to diagnostic errors.

SUMMARY

So what are clinicians to do? Analytical normative approaches to diagnostic reasoning such as those discussed in this article may be too time consuming, cumbersome, and impractical to use for every clinical encounter. Although most of the time heuristic thinking allows clinicians to work quickly and effectively, it may also lead to delayed or missed diagnoses. Is there a way to balance these trade-offs and use a combination of these approaches thoughtfully in actual clinical practice?

Indeed, Croskerry[17] argues that both the processes are essential to the clinician. Croskerry divides diagnostic reasoning strategies into System 1 and System 2 approaches. System 1 thinking involves the fast, intuitive, and often-unconscious processes typified by heuristic thinking. System 2 thinking represents the slower more analytical thinking exemplified by the hypothetico-deductive reasoning model. Using the best of both the approaches and knowing when to use them may be the path to effective diagnostic reasoning.[17]

It can be understood that heuristic thinking is not necessarily unscientific or unsophisticated. Rather, as mentioned, it is a useful and essential tool in the actual clinical context. Yet, the limitations of heuristics must be acknowledged and understood. When using heuristics alone, even seasoned clinicians may commit diagnostic errors.[23] There is a growing literature on describing cognitive biases, but rigorous research into the effectiveness of debiasing strategies is still lacking. Although not yet evidence based, there are some steps that clinicians can take that will likely lead them in the right direction.

First, a comprehensive understanding of the full range of oral, dental, and craniofacial disorders is essential. Second, clinicians should become familiar with the types of cognitive biases that arise from heuristics and how the biases might affect patient care. Some excellent reviews have been written on the subject, and several books written for the lay public also explore this topic.[19,24,25] Simply being aware of the dangers of heuristics might allow clinicians to recognize and avoid cognitive biases when they occur.

Clinicians can also use certain cognitive habits that might reduce the effect of some cognitive biases. Just as surgical time-outs and checklists have been shown to reduce errors, at the end of each clinical assessment, asking oneself "What else could this be?" is a type of cognitive time-out that might result in reduced incidence of diagnostic errors.[19,26] The clinician should be prompted when the information obtained in a case does not fit the initial diagnostic impression. In such a situation, the astute clinician should pause and use more analytical, stepwise, and rigorous approaches. As seen in case 4, considering disease outside the oral cavity may sometimes lead to the correct diagnosis. Thus, the hypothetico-deductive reasoning model is a strategy to be used not only by novices but also by experienced clinicians, when a given clinical presentation is vague, complex, or otherwise challenging.

Most clinicians do not formally calculate bayesian analysis each time a test is ordered. However, basic understanding of the concepts of bayesian analysis enhances the practitioner's use and interpretation of those tests. Furthermore, for tests that are used routinely, the practitioner may wish to search the literature to gain familiarity with that test's performance characteristics (sensitivity, specificity, and likelihood ratios). Diagnostic errors might also be reduced in complex workups with the use of decision trees and emerging decision support tools, although these tools have limitations. Online evidence-based clinical information is also increasingly available and used to support point-of-care clinical decisions.[27]

It has been noted that traditionally, dental school curricula have tended to focus on procedural technique while de-emphasizing diagnostic skills.[28,29] Dental schools should include discussions on diagnostic reasoning and diagnostic errors in their formal curricula and increase emphasis on diagnostic skills development. Further research is needed on the nature of cognitive bias in the dental profession and the effectiveness of debiasing strategies. Until evidence that can more definitively guide practice is found, developing clinical habits that use the benefits of heuristics, while relying on a more logical and analytical approach when necessary, will likely lead to more timely and accurate diagnoses and improved patient care.

ACKNOWLEDGMENTS

The authors wish to thank Dr Herbert Chase of Columbia University for his thoughtful comments on this article.

REFERENCES

1. Kassirer JP. Diagnostic reasoning. Ann Intern Med 1989;110:893–900.
2. Von Neumann J, Morgenstern O. Theory of games and economic behavior. Princeton (NJ): Princeton University Press; 1944.
3. Stempsey WE. Clinical reasoning: new challenges. Theor Med Bioeth 2009;30: 173–9.
4. Pauker SG, Kassirer JP. Decision analysis. In: Bailar JC, Mosteller F, editors. Medical uses of statistics. Waltham (MA): Massachusetts Medical Society; 1992. p. 159–78.
5. Sackett DL, Haynes RB, Guyatt GH, et al. Clinical epidemiology. A basic science for clinical medicine. Boston: Little, Brown; 1991.
6. Kositbowornchai S, Nuansakul R, Sikram S, et al. Root fracture detection: a comparison of direct digital radiography with conventional radiography. Dentomaxillofac Radiol 2001;30(2):106–9.
7. Waymack MH. Yearning for certainty and the critique of medicine as "science". Theor Med Bioeth 2009;30:215–29.
8. Berner ES, Graber ML. Overconfidence as a cause of diagnostic error in medicine. Am J Med 2007;121:s2–23.
9. Kahneman D, Slovic P, Tversky A. Judgment under uncertainty: heuristics and biases. Cambridge (UK): Cambridge University Press; 1982.
10. Patel V, Groen GJ. Knowledge-based solution strategies in medical reasoning. Cognit Sci 1986;10:91–116.
11. Elstein AS, Schulman LS, Sprafka SA. Medical problem solving: an analysis of clinical reasoning. Cambridge (MA): Harvard Univesity Press; 1978.
12. Schmidt HG, Norman GR, Boshuizen HP. A cognitive perspective on medical expertise: theory and implication. Acad Med 1990;65:611–21.
13. Feltovich PJ, Barrows HS. Issues of generality in medical problem solving. In: Schmidt HG, De Volder ML, editors. Tutorials in problem-based learning: a new direction in teaching the healthy professions. Assen (The Netherlands): Van Gorcum; 1984. p. 128–42.
14. Charlin B, Boshuizen HP, Custers EJ, et al. Scripts and clinical reasoning. Med Educ 2007;41:1178–84.
15. Neufeld VR, Norman GR, Feightner JW, et al. Clinical problem solving by medical students: a cross-sectional and longitudinal analysis. Med Educ 1981;15:315–22.
16. Cosmides L, Tooby J. Cognitive adaptations for social exchange. In: Barkow JH, Cosmides L, Tooby J, editors. The adapted mind: evolutionary psychology and

the generation of culture. Oxford (UK): Oxford University Press; 1992. p. 163–228.

17. Croskerry P. A universal model of diagnostic reasoning. Acad Med 2009;84(8): 1022–8.

18. Tversky A, Kahnemann D. Judgement under uncertainty: heuristics and biases. Science 1974;185:1124–31.

19. Croskerry P. The importance of cognitive errors in diagnosis and strategies to minimize them. Acad Med 2003;78(8):775–80.

20. Kohn L, Corrigan JM, Donaldson MS, editors. To err is human: building a safer health care system. Washington, DC: National Academy Press; 2000. p. 26–48.

21. Thomas EJ, Studdert DM, Burstin HR, et al. Incidence and types of adverse events and negligent care in Utah and Colorado. Med Care 2000;38:261–71.

22. Graber ML. Taking steps towards a safer future: measures to promote timely and accurate medical diagnosis. Am J Med 2008;121:S43–6.

23. Graber ML, Franklin N, Gordon R. Diagnostic error in internal medicine. Arch Intern Med 2005;165:1493–9.

24. Groopman J. How doctors think. New York: Houghton Mifflin; 2007.

25. Sanders L. Every patient tells a story: medical mysteries and the art of diagnosis. New York: Broadway Books; 2009.

26. Haynes AB, Weiser TG, Berry WR, et al. A surgical safety checklist to reduce morbidity and mortality in a global population. N Engl J Med 2009;360:491–9.

27. Available at: www.uptodate.com. Accessed June 20, 2010.

28. Glassman P, Chambers DW. Developing competency systems: a never-ending story. J Dent Educ 1998;62(2):183–96.

29. Crespo K, Torres J, Recio M. Reasoning process characteristics in the diagnostic skills of beginner, competent, and expert dentists. J Dent Educ 2004;68(12): 1235–44.

The Influence of Systemic Diseases on the Diagnosis of Oral Diseases: A Problem-Based Approach

Peter B. Lockhart, DDS[a],*, Catherine H.L. Hong, BDS, MS[a],
Denise E. van Diermen, MD[b]

KEYWORDS

- Stomatognathic diseases • Systemic disease
- Oral manifestations • Oral pain • Oral hemorrhage
- Medical history-taking

Although all dentists are taught about the importance of oral health to general health and that systemic disease can manifest in the oral cavity, time does not exist in the 4-year dental school curriculum to gain competency in these relationships. Nevertheless, all dentists must have skills in taking a medical history and an appreciation of oral findings that might have a systemic origin. These relationships between the mouth and the rest of the body are important for several reasons. First, the astute dental practitioner recognizes an abnormal oral finding and is aware that it could represent an oral manifestation of systemic disease. For example, enlarged gingiva usually represents a local, gingival or periodontal disease process, but this could also represent the first indication of a hematological malignancy from leukemic cell infiltration of the gingiva.[1] Exacerbation of periodontal disease in a patient with Type 1 diabetes is another example.[2,3] Second, history-taking and other information (eg, laboratory values, physician records and conversations) helps determine the extent to which patients' medical status allows them to tolerate stressful dental treatment (eg, the patient with unstable angina).[4,5] The vast majority of medical emergencies in the dental office are avoidable, and they usually stem from not knowing or taking into account the patient's medical history and current status, and how to modify the dental treatment

[a] Department of Oral Medicine, Carolinas Medical Center, PO Box 32861, Charlotte, NC 28232, USA
[b] Clinic for Medical-Dental Interaction, Department of Oral and Maxillofacial Surgery, Academic Center for Dentistry Amsterdam (ACTA), Gustav Mahlerlaan 3004, 1081 LA, Amsterdam, The Netherlands
* Corresponding author.
E-mail address: Peter.Lockhart@carolinas.org

Dent Clin N Am 55 (2011) 15–28
doi:10.1016/j.cden.2010.08.003
0011-8532/11/$ – see front matter © 2011 Elsevier Inc. All rights reserved.

plan accordingly.[6,7] Third, patients' dental status can directly affect their medical status. For example, edentulism results in an inability to masticate food and this has implications for a healthy diet, particularly with regard to nutrition in the elderly or otherwise compromised individuals. Also, patients' dental status may indirectly affect their medical status. For example, periodontal disease has been proposed as a risk factor for vascular disease.[8]

This article focuses on the identification of abnormal signs and symptoms in the oral cavity and the determination of those that have a systemic origin. It is imperative that clinicians are mindful of possible oral-systemic associations, because they can have an impact on the quality of patient care as mentioned earlier in this section.

APPROACHES TO THE DIAGNOSIS OF SYSTEMIC DISEASE

The traditional manner of teaching the relationships between oral and systemic disease is focused on an anatomic approach (eg, liver, bone marrow), a disease approach (eg, hepatitis, leukemia), or a drug approach (eg, cancer chemotherapy).

The organ approach focuses on an understanding of human physiology and what happens when organs and organ systems cease to function properly. Once this material is covered, the focus is on the implications for oral disease or abnormal oral findings. The organs most likely to manifest oral findings are the bone marrow, brain, endocrine system, heart, gastrointestinal tract, neuromuscular system, kidneys, and liver (**Table 1**). The most significant problem with the organ approach to oral disease is that patients do not necessarily know that they have organ disease or malfunction (eg, liver failure) and medical history-taking may not reveal its presence.

Table 1	
Organ and organ systems with oral manifestations	
Organ and Organ Systems	**Oral Manifestations**
1. Bone Marrow/ Hematology	Bleeding (petechiae, purpura, hematoma), delayed and/or poor healing, early loss of teeth, mucosal ulcerations, opportunistic infections (bacterial, fungal, viral), pallor
2. Heart	Cyanosis, referred cardiac pain (angina) to the mandible
3. Endocrine	Hyperpigmentation (Addison's disease), delayed eruption of teeth and enlarged tongue (hypothyroidism), periodontal disease and delayed or poor healing (diabetes)
4. Gastrointestinal	Halitosis, teeth erosion (gastroesophageal reflux disease), ulcerations (Crohn disease)
5. Liver	Bleeding (hematoma, purpura), discoloration of teeth (congenital liver disease), sweet musty odor, yellow pigmentation of mucosa (jaundice)
6. Neuromuscular	Difficulty with swallowing, mastication, speech, deviation of the tongue (facial palsy), drooling, poor oral hygiene and trauma due to poor control of musculature, taste changes
7. Brain	Enamel erosion from bulimia, aphthous ulcers, contribution to ANUG, poor oral hygiene, trauma from self-injurious behavior (eg, cheek/lip/tongue biting), TMD
8. Kidneys	Oral odor, radiographic changes in mandible and/or maxilla, pallor, taste changes, uremic stomatitis

Abbreviations: ANUG, acute necrotizing ulcerative gingivitis; TMD, temporomandibular disorder.

The disease approach to the relationship between the mouth and systemic disease is similar to the organ approach, focusing on the various diseases that occur with each organ or with multisystem problems. A long list of general disease categories have oral manifestations, including allergy, cancer, and immune suppression (**Table 2**). As with the organ approach, the problem with this approach is that patients do not always know that they have a systemic disease.

The organ and disease approach invariably include a discussion of drugs that have oral manifestations. For example, patients who are receiving intensive cancer chemotherapy or who are taking one of many psychotropic medications frequently have oral manifestations (**Table 3**).

The problem-oriented approach to identifying systemic diseases and disorders is the most useful from a practical and clinically relevant standpoint. Patients present to the dental office with a concern (subjective) about a change in their mouth or they are found by a member of the dental team to have a visible change in the hard or soft tissues (objective finding). There is a finite list of subjective concerns about the oral cavity that could represent a systemic disease or process. For example, patients can have altered sensation (eg, paresthesia) from a distant malignancy, mucosal ulceration from cancer chemotherapy, or gingival bleeding from an anticoagulant medication. Patients may present to the dental office completely unaware that they have a systemic disease and may be found to have a change in their oral soft tissues. There are various objective indicators of systemic disease, including changes in pigmentation from Addison disease or erythematous mucosa from a drug allergy. Finally, there is considerable overlap in the lists of subjective complaints and objective observations. For example, changes in color of a patch of mucosa (eg, leukoplakia after renal transplantation) may have been noticed by the patient or may first be noticed by a member of the dental team.

CASE 1

This 24-year-old non–English-speaking Hispanic man presented unaccompanied to the dental clinic of a large medical center with a chief complaint of nonhealing, bilateral ulcers on his tongue that had been present for about 2 weeks. He had moved to the United States recently from South America with his girlfriend. He denied any medical problems, medications, history of trauma, cough, smoking, or alcohol abuse. Squamous cell cancer, trauma, tuberculosis, and sexually transmitted diseases were on the differential diagnostic list, but all of these possibilities were considered unlikely given the medical history obtained through a translator. On a subsequent visit to the dental clinic 5 days later, the patient's girlfriend revealed that he had a long history of grand mal seizures. She stated that he refused to take his antiseizure medication and that he had multiple seizures in the past several weeks. He believed that epilepsy was a psychiatric illness, and his cultural background prevented him from admitting to a psychological or psychiatric problem. This case reveals the importance of persistence with the medical history to identify a systemic problem that is manifesting in the oral cavity **Figs. 1** and **2**.

CASE 2

This 41-year-old women presented to a hospital dental clinic with an asymptomatic swelling of her left lower face of 5-day duration. She was on a holiday visit to the United States from Canada. She was not being followed for any medical problems and she denied taking any medications or any history of trauma or toothache. The extraoral appearance was highly suggestive of an odontogenic abscess, but there were no

Table 2
Oral manifestations associated with systemic conditions

Oral Findings	Probable Causative Systemic Conditions
1. Altered Mucosa	Erythema and or ulceration: anemia, autoimmune disorders (eg, systemic lupus erythematosus, Behçet syndrome), gastrointestinal conditions (eg, Crohn syndrome), hypersensitivity reactions, medication-induced (eg, nicorandil), self-injurious behaviors (eg, chronic cheek biting), uremic stomatitis, vitamin deficiency
	Discoloration of oral mucosa: Addison disease, dermatologic diseases, heavy metal poisoning (eg, lead), liver disease, malignancy (eg, melanoma), medication-induced (eg, minocycline, quinolones, oral contraceptives), Peutz-Jeghers syndrome
	Oral blisters with or without ulceration: hypersensitivity reactions, vesiculobullous diseases, infections, self-injurious behaviors
	Pale oral mucosa: anemia, vitamin deficiency
	Xerostomia (subjective) or dry mucosa (objective): diabetes, medication-induced, Sjogren syndrome
2. Altered Sensation	Anemia, burning mouth syndrome, medication-induced, neuropathies (primary vs secondary causes), opportunistic infections, vitamin deficiency, xerostomia
3. Bleeding	Coagulopathies, medication or disease-induced
4. Musculature	Neurologic: nerve palsy, tardive dyskinesia, poor or defective muscle control causing drooling and accidental trauma
	Trismus: connective tissue diseases (eg, scleroderma), head and neck irradiation, neoplasm
5. Odor	Gastrointestinal conditions, respiratory infections, renal failure
6. Opportunistic Infections	Immunosuppression (eg, HIV/AIDS, hematologic malignancies), stress
7. Nondental Pain in the Head and Neck	Medication-induced (eg, vincristine), metastases, neoplasms, neuropathies (eg, primary vs secondary), referred pain (eg, cardiac, musculoskeletal, vascular), sickle cell crisis, temporomandibular disorders
8. Poor Healing	History of high-dose head and neck irradiation, immunosuppression, malnutrition, vitamin deficiency
9. Radiographic Changes in Maxilla and Mandible	Systemic conditions: Bone diseases: osteoarthritis, osteopetrosis, osteoporosis, Paget disease
	Connective tissue diseases: rheumatoid arthritis, scleroderma
	Genetic syndromes: cherubism, Gardner syndrome, Gaucher disease, Gorlin-Goltz syndrome, McCune-Albright syndrome, Papillon-Lefèvre syndrome
	Hematologic disorders: sickle cell anemia, Langerhans cell histiocytosis, thalassemia
	Immunosuppression: neutropenia, leukocyte adhesion disease
	Malignancies: Langerhans cell histiocytosis, multiple myeloma, metastases
	Primary or secondary hyperparathyroidism (from renal disease)
	Vascular conditions: carotid artery calcifications, intraosseous hemangioma, arteriovascular malformation

(continued on next page)

Table 2 (continued)	
Oral Findings	**Probable Causative Systemic Conditions**
10. Swelling	Soft tissue: acromegaly, amyloidosis, hemangioma, hypothyroidism, infection, lymphangioma, neoplasm, trauma Hard tissue: acromegaly, bone diseases (eg, Paget disease), hyperparathyroidism, infection, neoplasm, vascular lesions (eg, intraosseous hemangioma)
11. Teeth	Early loss of primary teeth: acrodynia, hypophosphatasia, histiocytosis X, immunosuppression (eg, cyclic neutropenia), juvenile-onset diabetes mellitus, neoplasms, nutritional deficiency, Papillon-Lefèvre syndrome Discoloration: genetic defects in enamel and dentine formation, hyperbilirubinemia, medication-induced (eg, tetracycline), porphyria Teeth erosion: eating disorders (eg, bulimia, gastroesophageal reflux disease) Rampant dental decay: hyposalivation

posterior teeth on the mandibular left side, clinically or radiographically. Further history-taking revealed that this swelling arose over a 1- to 2-hour period and that it had occurred once about 2 years earlier. The previous episode lasted about 7 to 10 days and disappeared in about the same amount of time as it arose. On further examination, a pulsatile sound could be heard through the face with a stethoscope. The patient was referred back to her physician in Canada for follow-up and was subsequently found to have an arteriovenous malformation. This case demonstrates the

Table 3
Common drugs that potentially induce oral manifestations

Drug Category	Oral Manifestations
1. Anticoagulants	Hematoma, purpura, risk of persistent bleeding after dental procedure or trauma, spontaneous oral bleeding with INR greater than the therapeutic range.
2. Antimicrobials	Black hairy tongue, discoloration of teeth (eg, tetracycline)
3. Antineoplastic Medications	Disturbances in craniofacial and dental development, jaw pain, opportunistic infections, stomatitis, taste changes, xerostomia
4. Antihypertensive Medications	Angioedema, lichenoid changes, stomatitis, taste changes, xerostomia
5. Antipsychotic Medications	Tardive dyskinesia, xerostomia
6. Antiseizure Medications	Bleeding tendencies, phenytoin-induced gingival hyperplasia, pernicious anemia (decreased absorption of vitamin B12)
7. Bisphosphonates (Oral and Intravenous)	Risk for jaw osteonecrosis
8. Calcium Channel Blockers, Cyclosporine, Phenytoin	Gingival enlargement
9. Herbal Medications	Bleeding tendencies (eg, ginger, gingko, garlic, ginseng)
10. Steroids	Moon facies, mucosal atrophy, opportunistic infections

Abbreviation: INR, international normalized ratio [TEE7].
Data from Refs.[18–20]

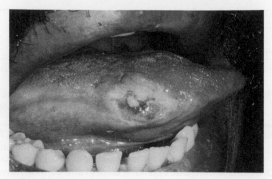

Fig. 1. Tongue ulcer of unknown origin.

importance of the medical history, in particular the HPI. If there had been teeth in the area, further suggesting an odontogenic abscess, and the swelling was incised, there would likely have been facial arterial bleeding as a result **Fig. 3**.

MEDICAL HISTORY-TAKING

Medical history-taking in general is a vitally important first phase in the evaluation of a new patient or one with a new oral finding or complaint on any subsequent visit (see **Figs. 1** and **2**). Before dental treatment can take place, the dentist has to determine if there are health problems that might alter the dental management of the patient. There are many medical diseases and disorders that can present with oral signs and symptoms, both subjective and objective. If a patient is aware of a medical diagnosis, the dentist can ask specific questions that target this issue and look for objective signs when performing the oral examination. In some situations, patients may be cognizant of a medical condition (eg, drug abuse) but may not want to disclose this aspect of their history (case 1). When patients are not aware of an oral or systemic condition, a thorough examination of the oral cavity might reveal an undiagnosed medical condition. This can be extremely important, for example, with oral signs or symptoms of human immunodeficiency virus (HIV)/AIDS, which may appear first in the mouth or may reappear if the HIV becomes unresponsive to antiviral therapy.[9] Also, the oral findings may strongly suggest an odontogenic problem but turn out to

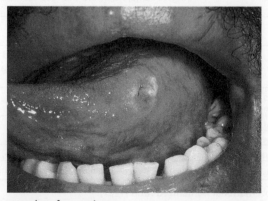

Fig. 2. Bilateral tongue ulcer from seizures.

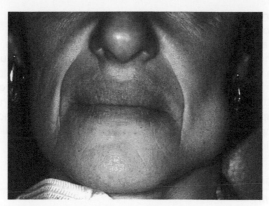

Fig. 3. Facial swelling caused by arteriovenous fistula.

have a nonodontogenic source that should be referred to a specialist for appropriate management (case 2).

A second reason for taking a medical history in the dental office is that medical disorders can result in medical urgencies and emergencies.[6,7] For example, patients with type 1 diabetes might experience a hypoglycemic episode during dental treatment, which may begin with a loss of consciousness and progress to a life-threatening situation. Also, patients with cardiovascular disease might experience angina during a stressful or painful dental appointment. When the dental team is aware of the medical conditions of their patients, appropriate precautions can be taken to avoid the vast majority of medical emergencies.

A third reason for taking a medical history is that certain patients need medication before invasive dental procedures. For example, some patients at risk of infective endocarditis are recommended for antibiotic prophylaxis before virtually all dental procedures.[10]

The medical history should initially be taken with the aid of a written form, to ensure that all medical conditions and medications that might be influenced by invasive dental treatment, or might be important for oral diagnosis, have been covered. This should then be followed by a verbal history-taking to ensure that important additional information has been gathered on positive or missing responses on the written form. Finally, patients should be questioned specifically about illnesses, hospitalizations, surgeries, medications, and allergies, because a negative response to all 5 of these items eliminate the majority of medical problems that arise during dental treatment.

Standard Medical History Format

Chief complaint
The reason for every nonroutine dental visit should be recorded in the patients chart, usually as the first line under the date.

History of present illness
The history of present illness (HPI) is critically important information as to the location and overall course of the problem that brought the patient to the office. The HPI usually has a description of some or all of the following: location, onset, duration, symptoms, severity, character, course, frequency, change in appearance, and past treatment for this problem. Some of this information may already be in the dental chart of the long-standing patient.

Past medical history

Past medical history (PMH) includes all past and current illness, hospitalizations, surgery, trauma, allergies, and medications. The date, location, and physician/surgeon for each hospitalization and/or surgery should also be included. Particularly important issues in the identification of oral manifestations of systemic disease include alcoholism, cancer, cardiovascular events, diabetes, and hepatic, renal, and psychiatric reasons for admission. Particularly important medications for oral manifestations include immunosuppressives, antibiotics, cardiac medications, and psychotropics. The PMH is also important for investigating whether the chief complaint (CC) is a manifestation of a previously diagnosed disorder.

Other Major Categories of Information Gathered

Review of symptoms

The review of symptoms (ROS) includes past or present problems with the major organs and organ systems. It usually begins with the head, eyes, ears, nose, and throat and goes on to cover the heart, lungs, liver, kidneys, and the neurologic and hematopoietic systems.

Social history

The social history (SH) includes questions pertaining to health habits, lifestyle, and nutrition, including the use of alcohol, tobacco, and other drugs, both prescription and recreational.

Family history

The family history (FH) is intended to cover all disorders and illnesses that may have implications for the patient, including cancer, cardiovascular disease, and inherited disorders.

Examination

The examination is conducted in the usual manner. In the case of lesions, for example, the focus is on location, size, number, color, depth, borders, palpation, odor, and so forth.

Assessment

The assessment is formulated from all the subjective and objective information gathered and may become a list of possible diagnoses in decreasing order of likelihood.

Plan

The plan is a list of things to be done, such as laboratory tests to be ordered, medications to be started and/or altered, and treatments to be instituted.

MAXILLOFACIAL INDICATORS OF SYSTEMIC DISEASE

Patient complaints (subjective information) or clinical findings (objective information) for a maxillofacial problem may represent a problem of systemic origin.

Subjective Indicators of Systemic Disease

Complaints or observations on the part of patients can be categorized into 9 groups: altered mucosa, altered sensation, bleeding, musculature, odor, poor healing, swelling, xerostomia, and problems with teeth.

Objective Indicators of Systemic Disease

In addition to the subjective indicators of systemic disease listed earlier, there are indicators that are objective alone, that is, patients are unlikely to be aware of these problems and they are identified by the dental health-care provider. These objective signs include altered mucosa, affected neuromusculature, psychiatric/psychological problems, and changes in the appearance of the teeth and/or radiographs.

Subjective and Objective Indicators of Systemic Disease

What follows is the list of subjective and objective indicators of systemic disease in alphabetical order (see **Table 2**).

Altered mucosa

Many disorders can alter the appearance of the oral mucosa, which can be lumped together under 2 major categories: color change and lesions. The appearance (surface texture, flat vs raised), size, intensity, location, and distribution of these changes (localized vs generalized) must be noted and the duration and frequency (if intermittent) included.

Color changes of the oral mucosa can be of a wide variety and are sometimes difficult to distinguish from what is normal for that patient (eg, pigmentation). As noted earlier, an important consideration is the determination of a localized change in color versus a generalized change. One of the more common color changes is a reddish (erythematous) color that is frequently associated with inflammation from a disease or an infection localized in the oral cavity, such as gingivitis. Oral infections can be divided into 3 varieties: bacterial, fungal, or viral. Infection in the oral cavity that arises in the absence of an obvious cause or that does not respond to conventional treatment should trigger concern for a systemic origin. For example, fungal infection, such as oral candidiasis, in the absence of the usual predisposing factors (eg, use of dentures, prolonged antibiotics or steroids; or xerostomia) might be caused by a failing immune system from AIDS, bone marrow failure (eg, aplastic anemia), hematologic malignancy, poorly controlled diabetes, nutritional deficiencies, stress, or any immunosuppressive disorder. Viral infections have a different clinical picture and can be represented by chicken pox, primary herpes or herpes zoster, or herpangina.

Color changes that have a systemic origin can be generalized erythema of the mucosa from a drug allergy or a more localized presentation, such as linear gingival erythema. Other color changes include a yellow discoloration from hepatitis, or an endocrine disorder in the case of a brownish tinge to the mucosa from Addison's disease. A localized bluish or black discoloration of the attached gingiva could represent heavy metal poisoning, and a generalized bluish coloration might represent cyanosis from a congenital heart defect. The classical black "hairy" (dorsal) tongue frequently results from prolonged systemic antibiotics, but it can have a range of colors as a result of the bacteriology of the elongated papillae. In rare cases, anemia can present with a generalized pallor to the oral mucosa. A whitish appearance can represent certain dermatologic conditions/diseases, such as discoid lupus erythematosus, HIV/AIDS, or vitamin deficiency. Other diseases and disorders can result in red patches (eg, Osler-Weber-Rendu) or red spots, such as petechiae from a very low platelet count.

Lesions of the oral mucosa from a systemic origin are numerous, and a complete description is beyond the scope of this article. They can have a localized or generalized appearance and can have various presentations. For example, historically, the dorsal tongue mucosa was important for diagnosing systemic disease, and it remains an important indicator of some disorders. Glossitis or an inflammatory change in appearance of the dorsal tongue can be an indication of an endocrine disturbance, such as diabetes, or a nutritional disorder from malnutrition, altered eating behavior, defective absorption, or vitamin deficiency. Other erythematous lesions may represent allergy, drug reactions, or medical therapy (eg, recent cancer chemotherapy or radiotherapy). Although unusual, ulcerations or oral erythema may represent a systemic cause, such as celiac disease, Crohn's disease, erythema multiforme, psoriasis, renal failure, systemic infections (eg, tuberculosis, venereal diseases, viral), systemic lupus erythematosus, and vesiculobullous diseases.

Altered sensation

Patients may complain of or have noted one of several changes in sensation associated with the oral mucosa, all of which can be grouped under burning, dysesthesia, pain, paresthesia, or taste.

A burning sensation is most often reflective of burning tongue or burning mouth syndrome. This disorder, by definition, does not result from factors such as vitamin deficiency, xerostomia, or diabetes, and they must be ruled out to arrive at a diagnosis of burning mouth. Characteristic or typical features of this disorder include a high incidence of a chronic, diurnal variation along with anxiety or depression.

Dysesthesia literally means *bad sensation*. Patients sometimes describe a burning, itching, or just unpleasant feeling. It can be caused by local factors, such as nerve damage, and by systemic disorders, such as Lyme disease, polyneuropathy from diabetes, or withdrawal from alcohol or drugs.

Pain or discomfort with the teeth or soft tissues of the mouth is another altered sensation that can have a nonoral origin. For example, the root apices of the maxillary posterior teeth are in close proximity to the maxillary sinus, and this should always be considered when there is a change in sensation that involves one or more of these teeth. A malignancy of the sinus cavity can penetrate the periapical tissues of the teeth and potentially mimic apical periodontitis or periodontal infection. Pain in the teeth from systemic origin can also reflect sickle cell crisis[11] or a side effect from some cancer chemotherapy agents.[12]

Another common pain entity in dental practice is temporomandibular joint disorder (TMD), which has typical and atypical presentations. Given that there is commonly a psychological component to this disorder, systemic considerations are important. In all situations, nonlocal or systemic conditions must be considered. For example, temporal arteritis can have significant overlapping symptoms with a typical TMD presentation (eg, temporal pain), but a failure to consider and rule out temporal arteritis could result in blindness.

Pain in the mandible, typically left sided, has long been identified with angina pectoris. The differentiation between anginal pain and an odontogenic source is usually straightforward, but failure to recognize the nonoral origin of mandibular pain could have profoundly negative consequences for the patient.[13]

Paresthesia is an abnormal sensation of the skin or mucosa, such as numbness or tingling, that has no objective cause. An onset of paresthesia in the maxillofacial region, in the absence of a local anesthetic injection, is a red flag for altered sensory nerve function, and this may relate to a process distant to the region. For example, cranial nerves can be involved with a tumor, resulting in entrapment or compression of the nerve. Paresthesia may also result from disease at a distant site, but with maxillofacial nerve involvement, such as metastatic cancer to the angle or body of the mandible.

The evaluation of a change or loss of taste can be complex, in that it involves the nasal passages and palate as well as different surfaces of the dorsal tongue. Loss or change of taste is closely associated with smell, and therefore a large proportion of complaints of taste change or loss are expected to be related to the loss or change of sense of smell. However, taste changes can also have their origin more distant from the tongue. For example, a tumor of the middle ear can result in change in taste (salty) to the anterior two-thirds of the tongue. Medications, such as cancer chemotherapeutic drugs, can cause transient changes, and radiotherapy to the midface or lower face can result in changes that are longer lasting. Given the complexity of the sense of taste, the dental practitioner should be aware that on occasion this altered sensation can result from a nonoral source and requires evaluation from an oral medicine or physician specialist.

Bleeding

Bleeding from the oral mucosa in the absence of even minor trauma is an unusual, if not a rare, phenomenon and needs to be thoroughly evaluated. History-taking is critical to the determination of cause of bleeding, in particular the FH, including current medications (eg, anticoagulants); alcohol intake history, previous history of bleeding, and duration of the bleeding episode; and liver, kidney or bone marrow disease. The first consideration is to determine if the bleeding is traumatic in origin or *spontaneous*. Spontaneous bleeding of the gingiva, that is, bleeding that begins in the absence of any trauma, is exceedingly rare. Spontaneous bleeding reported in the history or appearing during clinical examination is probably from minor manipulation of the gingiva. The next determination is to decide if the bleeding is from a local or distant source. For example, bleeding from minor trauma to the gingiva most often represents ulceration of the gingival crevicular tissue from gingivitis. Gingival bleeding in the absence of gingivitis or trauma is a more worrisome finding, and in the absence of a local cause, the practitioner needs to determine if the cause is a congenital (eg, hemophilia) or acquired phenomenon. Acquired causes are divided up into those entities that are either disease- (eg, leukemia) or medication-related.[14,15] Diseases that most commonly result in coagulopathies are of the bone marrow (eg, hematological malignancy, aplastic or thrombocytic anemia), liver (eg, viral hepatitis), and kidney (eg, uremia). Anticoagulants (eg, warfarin, antiplatelet drugs), chronic alcohol abuse, or vitamin deficiency (eg, scurvy) result in some degree of coagulopathy.

Neuromusculature

Neurologic disorders that manifest in the mouth include trauma, such as a tongue bite from seizures (see **Figs. 1** and **2**); palsy of part of the tongue and facial musculature due to paresis after cerebrovascular disorders or brain tumor; and tardive dyskinesia (involuntary and purposeless movements, such as grimacing, tongue protrusion, lip smacking, and puckering and pursing of the lips) from the use of antipsychotic medications. Inability to swallow, as can be seen in Parkinson disease, can manifest as drooling. Speech disorders can accompany neurologic disorders, making it difficult to understand the patient.

Odor

Odor that comes from the oral cavity can have systemic as well as local origin, for example acute necrotizing ulcerative gingivitis (ANUG).[16] Examples of a systemic origin include alcoholism, bronchiectasis, diabetes, gastrointestinal conditions (eg, gastroesophageal reflux disease), sinusitis, and uremia from kidney failure.

Poor healing

The oral cavity is almost unique in its ability to resist infection and the speed with which it heals, especially in young patients. Clinical experience gives practitioners the normal range of time during which the oral mucosa heals from a wound or infection.

Prolonged healing or failure to heal has always been a red flag for malignancy and may suggest the need for a biopsy or close monitoring. Prolonged healing may also suggest other systemic conditions such as immunosuppression from drugs, such as cancer chemotherapy, or bisphosphonates; aplastic anemia; or disease (eg, AIDS, cancer, diabetes). Nutritional compromise should also be considered.

Psychiatric/Psychological

Psychiatric illnesses and psychological problems are a common backdrop of oral and maxillofacial problems. One common set of problems, temporomandibular disorders, are often influenced by stressful situations. Other entities have long been thought to have a psychological component, such as ANUG, alteration of the dentition from certain eating disorders, chronic cheek chewing, exacerbation of lichen planus, grinding of teeth, and recurrent herpes labialis. Certain lesions in young children, such as condyloma acuminatum, soft palate petechiae, and torn labial frenum, have been reported to be indicators of abuse, and clinicians need to investigate further if there is a suspicion of this.

Radiographic changes

Various changes in bone (eg, multiple myeloma) and teeth (eg, tetracycline staining) might be noted by a member of the dental team. Radiographic changes may involve the lamina dura or periodontal ligament of the teeth or lucency, opacity, and trabeculae of the supporting bone. Systemic conditions that may cause radiographic changes in the maxilla or mandible include: bone diseases, connective tissue diseases, genetic syndromes, hematologic disorders, immunosuppressive conditions, malignancies, primary or secondary hyperparathyroidism, and certain vascular conditions.

Swelling

Swelling of the maxillofacial region and oral soft tissues is a common finding. As with facial swelling, oral swelling may have a systemic origin, including swelling of the salivary glands, lips, palate, tongue, and especially, the gingiva. The causes for swelling in this region may result from:

Allergy: Angioedema induced by medications, latex allergy.

Disease processes: Amyloidosis, autoimmune processes (eg, systemic lupus erythematosus), Wegener's granuloma, malignancies (eg, leukemia), orofacial granulomatosis.

Hormones: Pregnancy, birth control pills, overproduction of growth hormones, parathyroid and thyroid hormone problems.

Medications: Gingival hypertrophy induced by medications, such as calcium channel blockers, cyclosporine, and phenytoin.

Infections other than odontogenic and periodontal in origin: cat scratch disease, hemophilus influenza infection, mycobacteria infection, osteomyelitis, salivary gland infections.

Vascular: There are multiple causes for vascular-related swelling, some of which can be obscure but mimic common dental problems in appearance. For example, hospitalized patients with very low neutrophil counts after cancer chemotherapy can develop generalized facial swelling from vascular changes. An arteriovascular fistula can result in a facial swelling resembling a dental abscess (see **Fig. 3**). Vascular malformations and vascular tumors (eg, hemangiomas) are other vascular swellings that can occur in the head and neck region.

Vitamins deficiency: Vitamin C leading to scurvy.

Many diseases and disorders have gingival swelling as a manifestation. Patients who present with localized or generalized gingival enlargement without the typical appearance and behavior of gingivitis or periodontitis should trigger the clinician to think of systemic disease or drugs.

Teeth

The teeth have various changes in appearance that are indicators of a developmental or congenital condition, or systemic disorder, or a manifestation of a past problem. The result can be defective enamel or dentine formation, discoloration, eruption disturbances, mobility, and malocclusion. These changes can reflect disease, treatment for illnesses, and medications. For example, children who have had prolonged chemotherapy or radiotherapy that involves the jaws and developing teeth can have significant changes in appearance, such as defective formation of enamel and dentine, missing teeth and shortened roots. Discoloration of the teeth from renal failure is unusual, and the most common cause may be drug incorporation into the tooth structure during formation, as in tetracycline staining.

Xerostomia and dry mouth

Saliva is crucial to the maintenance of good oral health. It has antimicrobial, buffering, cleansing, digestive, and lubricating properties.[17] Some of the oral problems associated with lack of saliva include difficulty in chewing, speaking, and swallowing; difficulty with wearing removable dental prostheses; opportunistic infections; oral mucosal trauma; rampant dental decay; and taste changes. Common causes of xerostomia are dehydration and medications. The list of medications that can cause xerostomia is extensive (see **Table 3**). In some patients, the complaint of dry mouth may be an indication of a systemic condition, for example, diabetes mellitus or insipidus, and primary and secondary Sjögren syndrome.

SUMMARY

This article is by no means an exhaustive compilation of all the systemic conditions that manifest in the oral cavity. The primary goal is to provide dental clinicians with an appreciation of the importance of careful medical history-taking and thorough intra- and extraoral examinations, which together often provide valuable insight into patients' medical conditions, both diagnosed and undiagnosed.

REFERENCES

1. Gallipoli P, Leach M. Gingival infiltration in acute monoblastic leukaemia. Br Dent J 2007;203:507–9.
2. Nesse W, Linde A, Abbas F, et al. Dose-response relationship between periodontal inflamed surface area and HbA1c in type 2 diabetics. J Clin Periodontol 2009;36:295–300.
3. Salvi GE, Carollo-Bittel B, Lang NP. Effects of diabetes mellitus on periodontal and peri-implant conditions: update on associations and risks. J Clin Periodontol 2008;35:398–409.
4. Roberts HW, Mitnitsky EF. Cardiac risk stratification for postmyocardial infarction dental patients. Oral Surg Oral Med Oral Pathol Oral Radiol Endod 2001;91: 676–81.
5. Thompson SA, Davies J, Allen M, et al. Cardiac risk factors for dental procedures: knowledge among dental practitioners in Wales. Br Dent J 2007;203:E21.

6. Girdler NM, Smith DG. Prevalence of emergency events in British dental practice and emergency management skills of British dentists. Resuscitation 1999;41: 159–67.
7. Muller MP, Hansel M, Stehr SN, et al. A state-wide survey of medical emergency management in dental practices: incidence of emergencies and training experience. Emerg Med J 2008;25:296–300.
8. Humphrey LL, Fu R, Buckley DI, et al. Periodontal disease and coronary heart disease incidence: a systematic review and meta-analysis. J Gen Intern Med 2008;23:2079–86.
9. Phelan JA. Oral manifestations of human immunodeficiency virus infection. Med Clin North Am 1997;81:511–31.
10. Wilson W, Taubert KA, Gewitz M, et al. Prevention of infective endocarditis. guidelines from the American Heart Association. a guideline from the American Heart Association Rheumatic Fever, Endocarditis and Kawasaki Disease Committee, Council on Cardiovascular Disease in the Young, and the Council on Clinical Cardiology, Council on Cardiovascular Surgery and Anesthesia, and the Quality of Care and Outcomes Research Interdisciplinary Working Group. Circulation 2007;116:1736–54.
11. Ali R, Oxlade C, Borkowska E. Sickle cell toothache. Br Dent J 2008;205:524.
12. McCarthy GM, Skillings JR. Jaw and other orofacial pain in patients receiving vincristine for the treatment of cancer. Oral Surg Oral Med Oral Pathol 1992;74: 299–304.
13. Kreiner M, Falace D, Michelis V, et al. Quality difference in craniofacial pain of cardiac vs. dental origin. J Dent Res 2010;89(9):965–9.
14. Lockhart PB, Gibson J, Pond SH, et al. Dental management considerations for the patient with an acquired coagulopathy. Part 1: coagulopathies from systemic disease. Br Dent J 2003;195:439–45.
15. Lockhart PB, Gibson J, Pond SH, et al. Dental management considerations for the patient with an acquired coagulopathy. Part 2: coagulopathies from drugs. Br Dent J 2003;195:495–501.
16. Quirynen M, Dadamio J, Van den Velde V, et al. Characteristics of 2000 patients who visited a halitosis clinic. J Clin Periodontol 2009;36:970–5.
17. Napenas JJ, Brennan MT, Fox PC. Diagnosis and treatment of xerostomia (dry mouth). Odontology 2009;97:76–83.
18. Guggenheimer J. Oral manifestations of drug therapy. Dent Clin North Am 2002; 46:857–68.
19. Cohan RP, Jacobsen PL. Herbal supplements: considerations in dental practice. J Calif Dent Assoc 2000;28:600–10.
20. Abdollahi M, Rahimi R, Radfar M. Current opinion on drug-induced oral reactions: a comprehensive review. J Contemp Dent Pract 2008;9:1–15.

Dental Caries and Pulpal Disease

Domenick T. Zero, DDS, MS[a],*, Andrea Ferreira Zandona, DDS, PhD[a],
Mychel Macapagal Vail, DDS[b], Kenneth J. Spolnik, DDS, MSD[b]

KEYWORDS

- Diagnosis • Dental caries • Pulpitis • Periapical pathosis

MODERN MANAGEMENT OF DENTAL CARIES

The current practice of dentistry remains weighted toward surgically treating the consequences of dental caries. The importance of accurately diagnosing dental caries has in the past been overshadowed by the need to restore the extensive damage to tooth structure. With the advent of widespread use of fluoride in developed countries, the prevalence, severity, and rate of caries progression have declined. Consequently, practitioners can adopt a more conservative approach and apply the principles of modern management of dental caries.[1] These involve detecting and assessing caries lesions at an earlier stage; determining the caries risk status of the patient; making a diagnosis if disease is actually present; establishing a prognosis; applying intervention strategies focused on preventing, arresting, and possibly reversing the carious process; and delaying restorative treatment until absolutely necessary (**Fig. 1**). Most studies have evaluated these aspects of caries management as independent processes rather than one system that impacts the long-term health of patients. Ultimately, the usefulness of a diagnosis has to be judged by whether it leads to better treatment decisions and health outcomes for the patient, and thus, other factors, such as the risk/benefit and cost/benefit to the patient as well as patient preferences, need to be considered (see **Fig. 1**).

Challenges of Caries Diagnosis

Unlike many medical diseases, the diagnosis of the early stages of dental caries is not informed by the patient's symptoms, and there is almost complete reliance on the clinical presentation (signs) of the disease.[2] As the disease advances, there can be symptoms of pain and sensitivity to hot, cold, and sweet substances. In its later stages, there can be severe debilitating pain requiring endodontic therapy or tooth extraction.

[a] Department of Preventive and Community Dentistry, Indiana University School of Dentistry, Oral Health Research Institute, 415 Lansing Street, Indianapolis, IN 46202, USA
[b] Department of Endodontics, Indiana University School of Dentistry, 1121 West Michigan Street, Indianapolis, IN 46202, USA
* Corresponding author.
E-mail address: dzero@iupui.edu

Dent Clin N Am 55 (2011) 29–46
doi:10.1016/j.cden.2010.08.010
0011-8532/11/$ – see front matter © 2011 Elsevier Inc. All rights reserved.

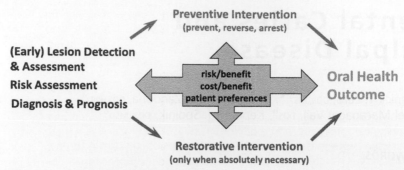

Fig. 1. Modern management of dental caries.

The detection of the signs and symptoms of dental caries is a component of and actually distinct from the caries diagnostic process, which leads directly to treatment decisions.[2] The caries diagnostic process must also include risk assessment at the patient and the tooth surface level and caries lesion activity assessment (**Fig. 2**). A degree of uncertainty exists when diagnosing the initial (noncavitated) caries lesions, because these early lesions may be active (progressing), inactive (arrested), or regressing (remineralizing). Therefore, a very important aspect of caries diagnosis is assessing the caries activity status of the actual caries lesion.[2–6] However, making an accurate clinical determination of caries lesion activity status is as challenging as it is important, and new technology-based methods to aid this assessment are needed.[5]

For several reasons, proportionally very little of a dentist's time is spent on the diagnostic process compared with physicians: (1) Reimbursement mechanisms in the United States reward operative and restorative treatment, whereas accurate diagnosis and disease prevention are not given high priority. (2) The diagnostic tools/procedures and codes for reimbursement are limited compared with medicine. (3) Dental schools

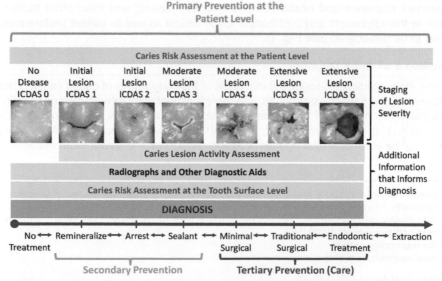

Fig. 2. Caries diagnosis and management system continuum as proposed by the International Caries Detection and Assessment System committee.

spend a substantial portion of curricular time on training to meet the technical demands of the practice of dentistry and proportionally very little on how to accurately diagnosis dental caries and manage it as a disease process, which leads to a continuing exacerbation of the problem.

Dentists vary widely when diagnosing dental caries, with agreement using traditional techniques ranging from poor to moderate (kappa values 0.30 to 0.60).[7] The consequences of misdiagnosis are inadequate treatment or overtreatment. Underdiagnosis leading to inadequate treatment can result in additional destruction of tooth tissue, pulpitis, toothaches, and tooth loss. However, dental caries is generally not an acute disease process but a chronic one that takes many years to progress in the postfluoride era. Overdiagnosis can lead to an unnecessary cascade of costly restorative treatment.[8] Based on data from the dental insurance industry, to maintain a single molar restoration placed in a 10-year-old patient reaches $2197 by age 79 years.[9] In many clinical situations, there is uncertainty about the diagnosis of caries. The paradigm in clinical practice and teaching needs to shift to surgical intervention being the last rather than first course of treatment considered by the dentist.

Role of Caries Risk Assessment and Caries Lesion Activity Assessment in the Diagnostic Process

As mentioned earlier, the caries diagnostic process includes 3 interactive components, namely, carious lesion detection, lesion activity assessment, and caries risk assessment, each informing the rest and all essential to making the best possible treatment decisions. Risk assessment of the patient and the tooth surface can help inform caries lesion detection and activity assessment as well as treatment decisions (see **Fig. 2**). Furthermore, caries lesion detection and activity assessment should help inform caries risk assessment, in that patients with detectable caries active lesions are at a minimum at moderate caries risk for future caries. Patients without clinically detectable caries active lesions may also be at moderate or high risk depending on recent changes in their risk factors/indicators.

Ideally, the goals are to identify patients at risk of developing caries before the disease process progresses to the point of expressing clinically and to use more aggressive primary preventive measures (professionally applied fluoride, preventive use of dental sealants). However, currently available caries risk assessment tools do not have sufficient accuracy to identify patients who eventually develop caries.[10,11] Based on available evidence, the best predictor of future caries remains past caries experience.[12,13] This suggests that in addition to recommending primary prevention measures (oral hygiene instructions, dietary advice, and recommending twice-daily fluoride dentifrice use) for all patients (see **Fig. 2**), dental professionals need to be vigilant during routine examinations to carefully detect dental caries at the earliest stages of the disease when secondary preventive measures (professionally applied fluoride, therapeutic use of sealants) are still possible and before surgical intervention is the only choice.

Incorporation of Caries Diagnosis into Patient Caries Management

Ultimately, the value of an accurate diagnosis is that it leads to the best possible treatment decisions and short- and long-term health outcomes. By combining the clinical presentation, including the severity of carious lesions and caries lesion activity assessment, with identifying caries risk factors of the patient and the tooth surface, a caries diagnosis can be made leading to the most appropriate treatment decision (see **Fig. 2**). This diagram is not intended to be prescriptive in recommending a particular level of intervention for each level of caries severity. The arrows pointing in both directions indicate that there is a treatment decision continuum that can be modified by risk factors of the individual patient and tooth surface, lesion activity status, and patient preferences.

Importance of Early Diagnosis of Pupal Pathosis

As the caries process progresses without some type of intervention, the pulp ultimately becomes involved. Being able to distinguish reversible pulpal symptoms resulting from caries from irreversible ones is paramount to deciding on the appropriate treatment. Knowing the early warning signs of pulpal and periapical disease certainly helps the practitioner decide on the most conservative treatment approach. The dental pulp is a resilient organ, and frequently, by removing the causative agent (caries), the pulp has the capacity to heal if there is no irreversible damage. By being alert to the clinical signs and symptoms associated with reversible and irreversible pulpal changes caused by caries, the practitioner can decide on the most appropriate treatment modality that potentially preserves the patient's natural dentition for a lifetime.

DIAGNOSING DENTAL CARIES

Dental caries is a dynamic disease process in which early lesions undergo many cycles of de- and remineralization before being expressed clinically. Its dynamic nature causes uncertainty about whether it is progressing, regressing, or in a state of equilibrium at any given point in time.[3,4] Once expressed clinically, caries can be detected by several detection methods, conventional (visual, radiographic) or newer technology-based (**Table 1**).[5]

Current approaches used in dental practice and still taught in most dental schools are inadequate for detecting and diagnosing dental caries at an early reversible/arrestable stage, and a new system to support the modern treatment paradigm is needed. One system that is gaining traction is the International Caries Detection and Assessment System (ICDAS), which is based on visual criteria. ICDAS was developed as a standardized evidence-based system[14] to assess severity stages of dental caries. It consists of 7 categories (0–6) to assess every tooth surface (see **Table 1**).[15] The application of this new system requires a major change in approach toward the clinical oral examination of the dentition. A quick look in the oral cavity for the purpose of detecting teeth requiring operative treatment is not adequate to properly manage the carious disease process. The correct application of ICDAS requires that all surfaces of each tooth are free of plaque and carefully examined under wet and dry conditions.[15,16] ICDAS has been shown to have good validity and reproducibility in several studies.[17–19] **Fig. 2** provides a summary of how ICDAS can be incorporated as part of a caries management system in which risk assessment of the patient, caries lesion severity and activity assessment,[5,6] and caries risk assessment of the tooth are used to establish the diagnosis and determine the most appropriate treatment.

Initial Lesion

The initial signs of dental caries involve surface softening, which cannot be detected by conventional visual or radiographic methods but could potentially be picked up by some technology-based methods, such as quantitative light-induced fluorescence (QLF), which has been reported to detect lesions as early as 35 μm deep.[20] Because the chemical composition of the carbonated hydroxyapatite is not uniform throughout the enamel, these variations result in varying enamel solubility.[21] Thus, the caries

Table 1
Caries detection tools

	Sound (No Disease)	Subclinical Caries	First Clinical Signs of Caries (Initial)	Established Caries (Moderate)	Severe Caries (Extensive)
ICDAS Codes[15-19]	0	0	1 + 2	3 + 4	5 + 6
X-ray[22,36,66-68]		Not detectable	Detectable on proximal surfaces	Detectable	Detectable
Light-Induced Fluorescence[17,46-51,a]	Some false positives	Detectable	Detectable	Detectable	Not useful
Infrared Fluorescence[52-57,b]		Not detectable	May detect some lesions on occlusal and smooth surfaces	Detectable	Detectable
Infrared Fluorescence Combined with Photothermal Radiometry[61-63,c]		Possibly detectable	Detectable	Detectable	Detectable
Transillumination[64-67,d]		Not detectable	Detectable on approximal surfaces and, in some lesions, occlusal surfaces	Detectable	Detectable
AC Impedance Spectroscopy[68-72,e]		Not detectable	Detectable	Detectable	Detectable

Abbreviations: AC, alternating current; ICDAS, International Caries Detection and Assessment System.
[a] Only Occlusal and smooth surfaces, limited data on root caries, caries around restorations and deciduous teeth.
[b] Occlusal, smooth, and proximal surfaces; limited data on deciduous teeth, root caries, and secondary caries.
[c] All surfaces, however, very limited data available only in vitro for occlusal surfaces, root caries, and smooth surfaces.
[d] Approximal and occlusal surfaces; very limited data available for secondary caries or deciduous teeth.
[e] All surfaces; very limited data available.

process starts in the most acid-soluble sites on the tooth surface, leading to small defects (increased porosity) allowing biofilm acids to diffuse below the surface and demineralize the more soluble subsurface tooth structure.

At the individual patient level, even teeth with ICDAS score 0 may be in need of primary preventive intervention (topical fluoride, preventive use of sealants) if caries risk factors/indicators suggest the patient is at risk of future disease. The first visual sign of dental caries as described by ICDAS is ICDAS score 1. These lesions are observed visually only after the enamel surface is dried for a few seconds. At this stage, histologically the early enamel lesions are limited to the outer enamel layer.[22] These lesions first appear as white spots and are sometimes called incipient lesions, white spot lesions, or even demineralization or decalcification areas. The lesion forms a conical shape, with the tip of the cone facing the enamel surface and the base facing the dentin.[23] Enamel lesions tend to progress in the direction of the enamel prisms; thus, the format of the lesion changes according to its location.[24] There is dissolution of the outermost surface of the enamel. The acid can attack the enamel rods or in between the enamel rods, causing an enlargement of intercrystalline diffusion pathways.[25] Carbonate and magnesium are first solubilized, followed by calcium and phosphorus solubilization and dissolution of developmental irregularities.[25,26]

The 4 distinct stages of porosity in carious enamel lesions[27,28] are associated with the 4 zones of the early enamel lesion: the surface zone, body of the lesion, dark zone, and primary translucent zone.[29] The surface zone is relatively intact, with a 1% pore volume (compared with 0.1% of sound enamel).[27,28] The body of the lesion, triangular in shape, has a 5% to 25% pore volume.[27,28] The dark zone pore volume is 2% to 4%, and the translucent zone, present in 50% of the lesions, has a pore volume of 1% to 4%.[27,28] The porosity of these early lesions is filled with water, and therefore, when the surface is wet, the difference in the refractive indices of water and air is not seen. However, when the surface is dried, water is replaced by air and the lesion is revealed.[23] The difference in diffraction coefficients of air and water, a physical phenomenon, results in the observed white color.[24] At this stage, the demineralization has not reached the dentin; however, in some instances, a reaction to the injury can be observed by the deposition of minerals in the dentinal tubules, referred to as tubular sclerosis.[30,31] Tubular sclerosis can be observed even before the bacterial invasion occurs into dentin and is not the lesion spreading laterally.[24] This is stimulated by the presence of the biofilm as a defense mechanism from the pulp-dentin complex.[32]

As the lesions further advance in the enamel, changes can be observed through the whole thickness of the enamel and sometimes affect the outer surface of the dentin (ICDAS 2). Optically and chemically, the changes observed in these lesions are the same as those seen in early enamel lesions. However, the changes are more pronounced and can be seen with the naked eye, even when saliva is coating the enamel surface. Histologically, this can be observed as complete dissolution of the thin perikymata overlapping areas corresponding to developmental irregularities (Tomes' processes, pits, and focal holes),[25,26] and there is greater enlargement of the intercrystalline spaces. At this stage, the increased permeability of enamel to acid and various other chemical stimuli leads the dentin-pulp complex to respond by increasing the activity of odontoblasts, which are stimulated to form a tertiary dentin matrix (reactionary dentin). The result may be retraction of their processes and an increase in collagen deposition in the periodontoblastic process space. In advanced enamel/early dentin lesions, color change is seen as a brown tint in the underlying dentin.

Moderate Lesion

When the lesions progress to the point of breaks occurring in the continuity of the enamel surface, forming microcavitations, they are referred to as ICDAS 3. This is a critical stage in the caries process, because once cavitation occurs, bacteria can easily invade the dentin,[24] quickening the process without allowing time for dentinal reaction to occur.[33] Nonsurgical treatment of this stage of caries is still possible, and sealants should be considered as a treatment option depending on individual patient factors (see **Fig. 2**).

In more advanced lesions (ICDAS 4), the lesion spreads along the dentino-enamel junction (DEJ) while destroying the mantle dentin. As the dentin is demineralized, it provides less support for the overlying enamel.[23] These lesions may be non-or micro-cavitated. The enamel has the same characteristics as in the advanced enamel lesions.

Extensive Lesion

As the lesion advances, bacteria invade the DEJ leading to an enlargement of the gap between enamel and dentin. The lesion become cavitated, when the enamel surface collapses, exposing the dentin (ICDAS 5 and 6). This cavitation fills with food debris and saliva.[23] The area where the bacteria are in direct contact with the dentin forms a leatherlike demineralized zone. The rate of carious lesion progression is reflected in the appearance of the peritubular zone, which is very thin or missing if the lesion progresses quickly. However, if the lesion expands slowly, sclerotic tubules form at the base of the lesion. The sclerotic tubules contain reprecipitated nonapatitic calcium phosphate.[34.] Bacterial acids demineralize the dentin and expose the extracellular matrix, which is subsequently degraded by matrix metalloproteinases found in the saliva and the dentin itself.[34,35] At this stage, the enamel surrounding the dentin has the characteristics of an advanced enamel lesion. Advanced lesions become darker brown or even black as they advance in severity.

Radiography

Radiography has been the primary detection method of established proximal caries.[36] As the carious process proceeds, the mineral content of enamel and dentin decreases, which decreases the attenuation of the x-ray beam as it passes through the tooth; a lesion is then detected by an increase in radiolucency.[36] To detect proximal lesions, the x-ray beam must go through normal tissue before it passes through the lesion and out through normal tissue again. Therefore, at least one-third to one-half of the hard tissue must be affected by the caries process for the lesion to be detected radiographically. Dental radiographs are useful in detecting larger, more advanced, and possibly cavitated lesions (ICDAS scores 2–6 on proximal surface and ICDAS scores 4–6 on occlusal surfaces, although some ICDAS scores 2–3 are detectable).[23] However, because of the limited image resolution and poor contrast of early carious lesions, radiographs are insensitive in detecting early-stage dental decay.[37] New imaging technologies and more sensitive techniques are required in the early detection of such lesions.[38]

Newer Technology-Based Caries Detection Methods

A wide range of technology-based methods can detect dental caries, and their use is recommended as diagnostic adjuncts.[5] These methods are more useful in the early and moderate stages of the dental carious process (ICDAS 1–4), because with increasing severity of the lesion, the visual signs become more apparent and thus reduce the need for additional tools. Although, in the authors' knowledge, no technology available can determine the activity status of the lesions in one visit, these tools can aid visual detection, diagnosis, and risk assessment. Several methods are currently marketed in the United States for caries detection, most being based on optical properties (Midwest Caries I.D., DENTSPLY Professional, Des Plaines, IL, USA; Microlux Transilluminator, AdDent Inc., Danbury, CT, USA), including fluorescence properties (DIAGNODent, KaVo, Charlotte, NC, USA; FluoreCam, Daraza, Noblesville, IN, USA; Inspektor Pro, InspeKtor Dental Care, Amsterdam, The Netherlands; Spectra Caries Detection Aid, Air Techniques Inc., Melville, NY, USA; The Canary System, Quantum Dental Technology, Toronto, Canada) and alternating current impedance spectroscopy (CariesScan PRO, CariesScan Ltd, Dundee, UK). Several reviews of these methods address principles and performance.[5,39–43]

Basically, demineralization of dental enamel causes scattering of light photons leading to optical disruption,[41,44] which can then be measured by detecting reflectance (Midwest Caries I.D.), a combination of luminescence and heat (The Canary System), differences in light transmission (Microlux), or impedance (CariesScan, PRO). Fluorescence systems are based on the difference in fluorescence observed between sound and demineralized enamel,[45] which is greater when the enamel is illuminated by light in the blue-green range (488 nm).[46–48]

In summary, fluorescence-based systems using light in the blue range (488 nm) have been reported to detect very early lesions,[20] smaller than visual examination is able to detect, and a greater percentage of noncavitated lesions than visual examination can detect.[49] This system has been investigated for its use on smooth and occlusal surfaces as well as for caries around restorations and root caries.[49–52] The lesions detected with these fluorescence methods range from ICDAS scores 1 to 4, sensitivity being higher than other methods at the lower end of the spectrum (ICDAS 1–2); however, this is at the expense of specificity (thus a high number of false positives).[53] The vast majority of the data published use the QLF Inspektor Pro software for analyses of the images, and it is not clear if the other systems have the same performance when different software is used for image analysis. However, because of the concerns regarding the noise caused by subclinical lesions that can be detected by QLF, there are reports combining the methodology with a clinical method without using the analyses aspect of the system.[19] Methods based on fluorescence at the infrared range (655 nm wavelength; DIAGNODent) have greater sensitivity for lesions deeper into enamel and dentin (ICDAS 2–4).[54–58] For caries around restorations, this can lead to many false positives.[59] The recently introduced Midwest Caries I.D. and the Canary System also use the near infrared laser light. The Midwest Caries I.D. is based on detecting changes in reflectance from sound enamel to demineralized enamel. Two published abstracts[60,61] indicate that this system was able to detect lesions at D3 level (caries in enamel and dentin) and performed better for detection of occlusal caries than proximal caries. On root caries, the system had sensitivities of 0.73 to 0.86 but did not perform better than ICDAS examinations.[62] The Canary System is based on analyses of luminescence and thermal behavior of the emitted infrared photons (noncontacting frequency-domain photothermal radiometry and frequency-domain luminescence). Published data[63–65] indicate that the sensitivity at the D2 threshold (caries in enamel only) is 0.81, whereas specificity is 0.87 for occlusal caries.

Transillumination methods (ie, Microlux) have at least the same sensitivity and specificity as bite-wing x-rays for detecting approximal and occlusal caries, achieving better performance for lesions into dentin.[66–69] Impedance (CariesScan PRO) is able to detect lesions on approximal and occlusal surfaces,[70] but limited data are available.[71–74]

DIAGNOSING PULPAL PATHOSIS

Dental caries is the most common cause of pulpal disease. As the carious process advances, the pulp undergoes various morphologic and histologic changes. Pulpal disease induced by dental caries can occur before bacteria actually invade the pulp. The earliest pulpal changes occur in the odontoblastic layer. These changes include a reduction in the number and size of odontoblasts and a loss of the pulpodentinal membrane.[75] These morphologic alterations are a change from all columnar cells to flat or cuboidal cells in the odontoblastic layer. In most cases, these odontoblastic changes precede inflammatory changes in the subodontoblastic region. Along with these changes in the odontoblastic layer, a calciotraumatic line develops between the pulp and primary dentin. Miller and Massler[76] suggest that this calciotraumatic line may be less permeable than normal dentin to noxious stimuli from carious lesions. This decrease in dentinal permeability may be due to a reduction in the number of dentinal tubules and/or a decrease in luminal diameter as a result of increased amounts of peritubular matrix.[77]

Torneck[78] states that the initial inflammatory response of the dental pulp to caries is primarily a mononuclear one, in which the dominant cells are lymphocytes and plasma cells. Therefore, it seems that the initial pulpal inflammatory response to dentinal caries is an immunologic phenomenon mediated by substances produced by the carious process. These substances can gain access to the pulp through the dentinal tubules before any microorganisms infect the pulp. These immunologic reactions could be an immune complex-mediated or delayed type of hypersensitivity.[79]

Massler[80] reported that enamel caries in newly erupted teeth produced inflammatory changes in the odontoblastic layer and not the subodontoblastic tissues. In adults with enamel lesions, Massler[80] did not find any inflammation within the pulp. Therefore, the inflammatory process in the pulp seems to be more prevalent in younger teeth with larger dentinal tubules than more mature teeth with fewer more occluded dentinal tubules.

Reeves & Stanley[81] found that bacteria needed to be within 1.1 mm of the pulp before significant inflammatory changes were observed in the pulp. They also observed that once the carious lesion was within 0.5 mm of the pulp, the degree of pathoses increased. However, evidence of irreversible pathosis was not observed until the reparative dentin was invaded.

In the early stages of pulpitis, there is increased vascularity with the proliferation of small vessels, characteristic of a chronic inflammatory response. However, once the carious lesion penetrates deeper into the primary dentin or invades the reparative dentin, more inflammatory cells appear and neutrophils begin to emerge from the surrounding venules. As the population of neutrophils increases, lysosomal enzymes are released, which play a significant role in the digestion of phagocytized bacteria. These enzymes assist in removing bacteria and also contribute to the destruction of pulp tissue, because they do not discriminate between harmful agents and host tissue. This leads to abscess formation and an increase in clinical symptoms.

Pulpal and Periapical Diagnostic Terminology and Associated Clinical Symptoms

In 2009, the American Association of Endodontists revised their diagnostic terminology to reflect these pathologic changes seen in the pulp as a result of caries or trauma. Although histologic findings may indicate unhealthy pulp, clinical tests may result in normal findings.[82] For example, an inflamed pulp that is characterized by inflammatory cells may test normal, clinically, if there is some residual normal tissue. Treatment of the tooth with root canal therapy is dictated by the vitality of the tooth, the patient's symptoms, and the radiographic presentation. Vitality, but not health or disease of the pulp, is tested by cold using ice sticks, tetrafluoroethane spray, carbon dioxide snow, and/or electric pulp test (EPT).[83] Lin and Chandler[84] reported higher than 80% accuracy of pulp vitality test when thermal test and EPT techniques are used. A tender response to percussion by the handle of a mouth mirror indicates some degree of periapical inflammation that may be caused by malocclusion, trauma, periodontal disease, or pulpal disease that has reached the periapical tissues. The following definitions describe the state of the pulp and periapical tissues through the use of clinical objective findings, radiographic interpretation, and patient's subjective symptoms.

The diagnostic nomenclature is divided into pulpal and periapical terminology (**Tables 2** and **3**).[85,86] Pulpal diagnosis can be classified as normal pulp, reversible pulpitis, irreversible pulpitis, or pulp necrosis. Periapical diagnosis is classified as normal apical tissues, symptomatic apical periodontitis, asymptomatic apical periodontitis, acute apical abscess, chronic apical abscess, or condensing osteitis. A healthy pulp is characterized by a short nonlingering response to cold that subsides almost immediately when the stimulus is removed. In reversible pulpitis, the pulp has mild inflammation caused by caries, trauma, or defective or recent restorations. A cold test elicits a quick and sometimes sharp response, but the discomfort does not linger. The patient does not report a history of spontaneous pain, and once the cause of the inflammation is removed, the pulp returns to a healthy state and does not require root canal therapy.[85,87] Percussion does not elicit discomfort, and radiographic images do not show periapical pathosis in both normal pulp and reversible pulpitis.

Irreversible pulpitis and pulp necrosis are 2 pulp conditions that have further evolved into a more advanced state of pulpal disease that requires root canal therapy or extraction.[88] Irreversible pulpitis, the precursor of pulpal necrosis if untreated, is categorized as symptomatic or asymptomatic.[85,89,90] Berman and Hartwell[85] state that "the acutely inflamed pulp is symptomatic and the chronically inflamed pulp is asymptomatic." In contrast to asymptomatic irreversible pulpitis, symptomatic pulpitis is characterized by spontaneous, lingering pain, and the symptoms can be duplicated when the patient is subjected to the cold test. Percussion sensitivity may develop if the inflammatory process has progressed to the periapical tissues.[91] Radiographic examination may reveal a thickening of the periodontal ligament (PDL) in advanced state, but otherwise it appears normal.[85,91]

As the pulp destruction continues and pulpitis is left untreated, a necrotic pulp results. Clinical symptoms may range from no pain to severe pain depending on the extent of periapical inflammation. Total necrosis of the pulp elicits no response to cold or EPT. Compared with other histopathologic presentations, necrosis correlates predictably with a negative response to cold; however, some studies refute this, because of the partial tissue that may still be present.[85,91] Radiographs vary, revealing a normal periapex to large periapical radiolucency; the percussion test may elicit discomfort.

According to the revised diagnostic terminology, the category of *normal apical tissues* refers to teeth that do not respond to pain on percussion or palpation and to radiographs showing evidence of an intact lamina dura and uniform PDL.[90] Once pulpal inflammation reaches the apical tissues, pathologic changes can occur in the periradicular tissues. Periradicular pathoses range from slight inflammation to resorption of the periradicular bone. The severity of the irritant, the duration of the disease process, and the host response determines the extent of destruction, usually mediated by nonspecific and specific immune reactions.[88,92] Symptomatic apical periodontitis results from pulpal inflammation into the periradicular tissues. Clinically,

Table 2
Diagnosis of pulpal pathosis

	Normal Pulp	Reversible Pulpitis	Irreversible Pulpitis (Asymptomatic)	Irreversible Pulpitis (Symptomatic)	Pulp Necrosis
Signs					
Patient History	No history of spontaneous pain	No history of spontaneous pain	None	Spontaneous pain	No pain to severe pain
Cold Test	Quick mild response to cold and does not linger	Quick and sometimes sharp response; discomfort does not linger	Quick and sometimes sharp response; discomfort does not linger	Exaggerated response to cold with lingering pain	No response
Percussion Sensitivity	Negative	Negative	Negative	May be positive	No response to exaggerated response
Radiographic Periapical Findings	Normal	Normal	Normal PDL or thickening of PDL Caries present	Normal PDL or thickening of PDL	Normal periapex to large periapical radiolucency

Abbreviation: PDL, periodontal ligament.

Table 3
Diagnosis of periapical disease

	Normal Periapical Tissues	Symptomatic Apical Periodontitis	Asymptomatic Apical Periodontitis	Acute Apical Abscess	Chronic Apical Abscess
Patient History of Symptoms	None	Pain when biting	None	Extreme pain when biting	Usually none
Vitality Tests	WNL	Usually no response to vitality tests	No response to vitality tests	No response to vitality Tests	No response
Percussion	None	Positive	None to slight	Positive	None to slight
Palpation	None	May or may not be positive	WNL	Positive	None to slight with sinus tract present
Radiographic Findings	Normal	Widened PDL space to PAR	PAR	Widened PDL space to PAR	PAR

Abbreviations: PAR, periapical radiolucency; PDL, periodontal ligament; WNL, within normal limits.

patients may experience moderate to severe spontaneous pain or pain on percussion and biting. Radiographs may show a widened PDL and an intact lamina dura. Histologic features include polymorphonuclear (PMN) leukocytes and macrophages, and possibly, liquefaction necrosis in small areas of the pulp. At this point, the pulp may still test vital with cold test and EPT. Asymptomatic apical periodontitis can progress into symptomatic apical periodontitis. By definition, the patient has no symptoms and teeth do not respond to the cold test or EPT and have an unremarkable response to percussion or palpation. Radiographic images may vary from a break in the lamina dura to a large periapical radiolucency. Histologic presentation would be consistent with a periapical granuloma or an apical cyst.[88] A variant of asymptomatic apical periodontitis is condensing osteitis, which represents an increase in trabecular bone as a response to a low-grade persistent irritation.[88] Histologically, condensing osteitis is characterized by a dense mass of lamellar bone surrounding regions of connective tissue, epithelium, and inflammatory cells.[93]

Acute apical abscess can be localized or diffuse, characterized by rapid onset, spontaneous pain and swelling; however, swelling does not occur if the abscess is confined to bone. Histologic features show localized liquefaction necrosis with abundant PMN leukocytes, debris, and accumulation of purulent exudates. Chronic apical abscess is a longstanding lesion that stems from a draining abscess, and it presents clinically as a sinus tract. The patient has little or no discomfort and usually has drainage from the associated sinus tract.[85,88,90] Sinus tracts may not be located on the overlying soft tissue of the offending tooth. Placement of a gutta-percha point into the tract helps identify the source of the infection.

SUMMARY

As more advanced approaches become available for managing dental caries as a disease process and maintaining pulp vitality, the need will increase for early and accurate diagnosis and monitoring of dental caries and pulpal/periapical pathosis. Although there have been some advances in new technologies to assist practitioners in detecting and assessing carious lesions, existing methods have limitations and, if not used properly, can lead to overtreatment.

Future advances in pulp testing procedures, perhaps directed more at blood flow than neural conduction, may lead to the detection of early pulpal changes that help direct more conservative approaches to treatment of carious lesions. The conebeam CT scanners would also enhance the diagnosis of periapical pathosis much sooner than conventional radiographic techniques, thus providing earlier intervention before the disease process exacerbates.

As the ability to diagnose dental disease improves, treatment approaches will become more conservative, leading to more preservation of natural tooth structure.

REFERENCES

1. Pitts NB. Modern concepts of caries measurement. J Dent Res 2004;83:C43–7.
2. Nyvad B. Diagnosis versus detection of caries. Caries Res 2004;38:192–8.
3. Nyvad B, Fejerskov O. Assessing the stage of caries lesion activity on the basis of clinical and microbiological examination. Community Dent Oral Epidemiol 1997; 25:69–75.
4. Zero DT. Dental caries process. Dent Clin North Am 1999;43:635–64.
5. Ferreira Zandona A, Zero DT. Diagnostic tools for early caries detection. J Am Dent Assoc 2006;137:1675–84.

6. Ekstrand KR, Zero DT, Martignon S, et al. Lesion activity assessment. Monogr Oral Sci 2009;21:63–90.
7. Bader JD, Shugars DA. Variation in dentists' clinical decisions. J Public Health Dent 1995;55:181–8.
8. Elderton RJ. Clinical studies concerning re-restoration of tooth. Adv Dent Res 1990;4:4–9.
9. Northeast Delta Dental. The true cost of a cavity. Available at: http://www.admin.state.nh.us/wellness/PDF/Resources/Dental%20True_Cost_of_a_Cavity.pdf. Accessed June, 2010.
10. Hausen H. Caries prediction - state of the art. Community Dent Oral Epidemiol 1997;25:87–96.
11. Hausen H, Kärkkäinen S, Seppä L. Application of the high-risk strategy to control dental caries. Community Dent Oral Epidemiol 2000;28:26–34.
12. Disney JA, Graves RC, Stamm JW, et al. The University of North Carolina Caries Risk Assessment study: further developments in caries risk prediction. Community Dent Oral Epidemiol 1992;20:64–75.
13. Zero D, Fontana M, Lennon AM. Clinical applications and outcomes of using indicators of risk in caries management. J Dent Educ 2001;65:1126–32.
14. Pitts N. "ICDAS"–an international system for caries detection and assessment being developed to facilitate caries epidemiology, research and appropriate clinical management. Community Dent Health 2004;21:193–8.
15. Topping GV, Pitts NB. Clinical visual caries detection. In: Pitts NB, editor. Detection, assessment, diagnosis and monitoring of caries. Basel (Switzerland), Karger: Monogr Oral Sci; 2009. p. 15–41.
16. ICDAS criteria manual: modified PDF version (2009) of criteria manual for the International Caries Detection and Assessment System (ICDAS II). Available at: http://www.icdasfoundation.dk/. Accessed June, 2010.
17. Ismail AI, Sohn W, Tellez M, et al. The International Caries Detection and Assessment System (ICDAS): an integrated system for measuring dental caries. Community Dent Oral Epidemiol 2007;35(3):170–8.
18. Mendes FM, Braga MM, Oliveira LB, et al. Discriminant validity of the International Caries Detection and Assessment System (ICDAS) and comparability with World Health Organization criteria in a cross-sectional study. Community Dent Oral Epidemiol 2010;38:398–407.
19. Ferreira Zandona AG, Santiago E, Eckert G, et al. The Use of ICDAS combined with QLF as a caries detection method. Caries Res 2010;44:317–22.
20. Ferreira Zandoná AG, Analoui M, Beiswanger BB, et al. An in vitro comparison between laser fluorescence and visual examination for detection of demineralization in occlusal pits and fissures. Caries Res 1998;32:210–8.
21. Robinson C, Shore RC, Brookes SJ, et al. The chemistry of enamel caries. Crit Rev Oral Biol Med 2000;11(4):481–95.
22. Ekstrand KR, Ricketts DN, Kidd EA. Reproducibility and accuracy of three methods for assessment of demineralization depth on the occlusal surface: An in vitro examination. Caries Res 1997;31(3):224–31.
23. Ekstrand KR, Ricketts DN, Kidd EA. Occlusal caries: pathology, diagnosis and logical management. Dent Update 2001;28(8):380–7.
24. Kidd EAM, Fejerskov O. What constitutes dental caries? Histopathology of carious enamel and dentin related to the action of cariogenic biofilms. J Dent Res 2004;83:C35–8.
25. Holmen L, Thylstrup A, Øgaard B, et al. Scanning electron microscopy study of progressive stages of enamel caries in vivo. Caries Res 1985;19:355–67.

26. Holmen L, Thylstrup A, Årtun J. Clinical and histological features observed during arrestment of active enamel carious lesions in vivo. Caries Res 1987;21:546–54.
27. Darling AL. Studies of the early lesion of enamel caries with transmitted light, polarised light and radiography. Braz Dent J 1956;101:289–97.
28. Darling AI. The selective attack of caries on the dental enamel. Ann R Coll Surg Engl 1961;29:354–69.
29. Silverstone LM. Structure of carious enamel, including the early lesion. Oral Sci Rev 1973;3:100–60.
30. Johnson NW, Taylor BR, Berman DS. The response of deciduous dentine to caries studied by correlated light and electron microscopy. Caries Res 1969;3: 348–68.
31. Stanley HR, Pereira JC, Spiegel EH, et al. The detection and prevalence of reactive and physiologic sclerotic dentin, reparative dentin, and dead tracts beneath various types of dental lesions according to tooth surface and age. J Oral Pathol 1983;12:257–89.
32. Bjørndal L, Thylstrup A. A structural analysis of approximal enamel caries lesions and subjacent dentin reactions. Eur J Oral Sci 1995;103:25–31.
33. Thylstrup A, Qvist V. Principal enamel and dentine reactions during caries progression. In: Thylstrup A, Leach SA, Qvist V, editors. Dentine and dentine reactions in the oral cavity. Oxford (UK): IRL Press; 1987. p. 3–16.
34. Chaussain-Miller C, Fioretti F, Goldberg M, et al. The role of matrix metalloproteinases (MMPs) in human caries. J Dent Res 2006;85(1):22–32.
35. Tjaderhane L, Larjava H, Sorsa T, et al. The activation and function of host matrix metalloproteinases in dentin matrix breakdown in caries lesions. J Dent Res 1998; 77(8):1622–9.
36. Dove B. Radiographic diagnosis of dental caries. J Dent Educ 2001;65(10): 985–90.
37. Ko A, Hewko M, Sowa M, et al. Early dental caries detection using fibre-optic coupled polarization-resolved Raman spectroscope system. Opt Express 2008; 16(9):6274–84.
38. Jones R, Huynh G, Jones G, et al. Near-infrared transillumination at 1310-nm for the imaging of early dental decay. Opt Express 2003;11(18):2259–65.
39. Bader JD, Shugars DA, Bonito AJ. Systematic reviews of selected dental caries diagnostic and management methods. J Dent Educ 2001;65(10):960–8.
40. Bader JD, Shugars DA. A systematic review of the performance of a laser fluorescence device for detecting caries. J Am Dent Assoc 2004;135(10):1413–26.
41. Pretty IA. Caries detection and diagnosis: novel technologies. J Dent 2006;34: 727–39.
42. Stookey GK. Quantitative light fluorescence: a technology for early monitoring of the caries process. Dent Clin North Am 2005;49(4):753–70.
43. Yang J, Dutra V. Utility of radiology, laser fluorescence, and transillumination. Dent Clin North Am 2005;49(4):739–52.
44. Angmar-Månsson B, ten Bosch JJ. Advances in methods for diagnosing coronal caries-a review. Adv Dent Res 1993;7(2):70–9.
45. Benedict HC. Notes on the fluorescence of teeth in ultra-violet rays. Science 1928;67(1739):442.
46. Alfano RR, Yao SS. Human teeth with and without dental caries studied by visible luminescent spectroscopy. J Dent Res 1981;60(2):120–2.
47. Bjelkhagen H, Sundström F, Ångmar-Månsson B, et al. Early detection of enamel caries by the luminescence excited by visible laser light. Swed Dent J 1982;6(1): 1–7.

48. Sundström F, Fredriksson K, Montan S, et al. Laser-induced fluorescence from sound and carious tooth substance: spectroscopic studies. Swed Dent J 1985; 9(2):71–80.

49. Kühnisch JI, Tranæus S, Hickel R, et al. In vivo detection of non-cavitated caries lesions on occlusal surfaces by visual inspection and quantitative light-induced fluorescence. Acta Odontol Scand 2007;65(3):183–8.

50. Feng Y, Yin W, Hu D, et al. Assessment of autofluorescence to detect the remineralization capabilities of sodium fluoride, monofluorophosphate and non-fluoride dentifrices. A single-blind cluster randomized trial. Caries Res 2007;41(5): 358–64.

51. Ando M, Gonzalez-Cabezas C, Isaacs RL, et al. Evaluation of several techniques for the detection of secondary caries adjacent to amalgam restorations. Caries Res 2004;38(4):350–6.

52. Pretty IA, Ingram GS, Agalamanyi EA, et al. The use of fluorescein-enhanced quantitative light-induced fluorescence to monitor de- and re-mineralization of in vitro root caries. J Oral Rehabil 2003;30(12):1151–6.

53. Ferreira-Zandoná AG, Stookey GK, Eggertsson H, et al. Clinical validation study of QLF at Indiana. In: Early detection of dental caries III: Proceedings of the 6th Annual Indiana Conference. Indianapolis: 2003, p. 237–52.

54. Lussi A, Hack A, Hug I, et al. Detection of approximal caries with a new laser fluorescence device. Caries Res 2006;40:97–103.

55. Shinohara T, Takase Y, Amagai T, et al. Criteria for a diagnosis of caries through the DIAGNOdent. Photomed Laser Surg 2006;24(1):50–8.

56. Goel A, Chawla HS, Gauba K, et al. Comparison of validity of DIAGNOdent with conventional methods for detection of occlusal caries in primary molars using the histological gold standard: an in vivo study. J Indian Soc Pedod Prev Dent 2009; 27(4):227–34.

57. Khalife MA, Boynton JR, Dennison JB, et al. In vivo evaluation of DIAGNOdent for the quantification of occlusal dental caries. Oper Dent 2009;34(2):136–41.

58. Costa AM, Paula LM, Bezerra AC. Use of Diagnodent for diagnosis of non-cavitated occlusal dentin caries. J Appl Oral Sci 2008;16(1):18–23.

59. Bamzahim M, Aljehani A, Shi XQ. Cinical performance of DIAGNOdent in the detection of secondary carious lesions. Acta Odontol Scand 2005;63(1):26–30.

60. Braun A, Kapsalis A, Jepsen S, et al. Approximal caries detection with a LED based device in vivo [abstract number 0142]. J Dent Res 2008;87(Spec Iss B). Available at: www.dentalresearch.org. Accessed August 10, 2010.

61. Krause F, Melner DJ, Stawirej R, et al. LED based occlusal and approximal caries detection in vitro [abstract number 0526]. J Dent Res 2008;87(Spec Iss B). Available at: www.dentalresearch.org. Accessed August 10, 2010.

62. Zeckel IN, Zandona AGF, Eckert GJ. Comparing ICDAS on root surfaces with non-conventional caries detection tools [abstract number 3362]. J Dent Res 2009; 87(Spec Iss A). Available at: www.dentalresearch.org. Accessed August 10, 2010.

63. Jeon RJ, Han C, Mandelis A, et al. Diagnosis of pit and fissure caries using frequency-domain infrared photothermal radiometry and modulated laser luminescence. J Can Dent Assoc 2004;70(7):470–4.

64. Jeon RJ, Hellen A, Matvienko A, et al. In vitro detection and quantification of enamel and root caries using infrared photothermal radiometry and modulated luminescence. J Biomed Opt 2008;13(3):034025.

65. Matvienko A, Jeon J, Mandelis A, et al. Dental biothermophotonics: a quantitative photothermal analysis of early demineralization. Eur Phys J Spec Top 2008;153: 463–5.
66. Côrtes DF, Ekstrand KR, Elias-Boneta AR, et al. An in vitro comparison of the ability of fibre-optic transillumination, visual inspection and radiographs to detect occlusal caries and evaluate lesion depth. Caries Res 2000;34:443–7.
67. Mialhe FL, Pereira AC, Pardi V, et al. Comparison of three methods for detection of carious lesions in proximal surfaces versus direct visual examination after tooth separation. J Clin Pediatr Dent 2003;28(1):59–62.
68. Peers A, Hill FJ, Mitropoulos CM, et al. Validity and reproducibility of clinical examination, fibre-optic transillumination, and bite-wing radiology for the diagnosis of small approximal carious lesions: an in vitro study. Caries Res 1993; 27(4):307–11.
69. Chesters RK, Pitts NB, Matuliene G, et al. An abbreviated caries clinical trial design validated over 24 months. J Dent Res 2002;81(9):637–40.
70. Huysmans MC, Longbottom C, Pitts NB, et al. Impedance spectroscopy of teeth with and without approximal caries lesions–an in vitro study. J Dent Res 1996; 75(11):1871–8.
71. Pitts NB, Los P, Biesak M, et al. Ac-impedance spectroscopy technique for monitoring dental caries in human teeth. Caries Res 2007;41(4):321–2 [abstract 153].
72. Pitts NB, Longbottom C, Ricketts D, et al. Hidden dentinal caries detection using a novel electrical impedance device [abstract number 2836]. J Dent Res 2008; 86(Spec Iss A). Available at: www.dentalresearch.org. Accessed August 10, 2010.
73. Los P, Longbottom C, Hall AF, et al. Ac-impedance spectroscopy technique for the detection of dental caries in human teeth. Caries Res 2007;41(4):296–7 [abstract 80].
74. Longbottom C, Hall AF, Czajczynska-Waszkiewicz A, et al. Caries detection by optimal clinical visual, radiographic, laser fluorescence and AC impedance spectroscopy techniques. Caries Res 2007;41:297 [abstract 81].
75. Bronnstrom M, Lind P. Pulpal response to early dental caries. J Am Dent Assoc 1965;5:1045–50.
76. Miller WA, Massler M. Permeability and staining of active and arrested lesions in dentin. Braz Dent J 1962;112:187–97.
77. Scott JN, Weber DF. Microscopy of the junctional region between human coronal primary and secondary dentin. J Morphol 1977;154:133–45.
78. Torneck C. A report of studies into changes in the fine structure of the dental pulp in human caries pulpitis. J Endod 1981;7:8–16.
79. Trowbridge HO. Pathogenesis of pulpitis resulting from dental caries. J Endod 1981;7:52–9.
80. Massler M. Pulpal reaction to dentinal caries. J Dent Res 1967;17:441–60.
81. Reeves R, Stanley HR. The relationship of bacterial penetration and pulpal pathosis in carious teeth. Oral Surg Oral Med Oral Pathol 1966;22:59–71.
82. Seltzer S, Bender IB, Ziontz M. The dynamics of pulp inflammation: Correlations between diagnostic data and actual histologic findings in the pulp. Oral Surg Oral Med Oral Pathol 1963;16:969–77.
83. Newton CW, Hoen MM, Goodis HE, et al. Identify and determine the metrics, hierarchy, and predictive value of all the parameters and/or methods used during endodontic diagnosis. J Endod 2009;12:1635–44.
84. Lin J, Chandler NP. Electric pulp testing: a review. Int Endod J 2008;41:365–74.

85. Berman LH, Hartwell CG. Diagnosis. In: Cohen S, Hargreaves KM, editors. Pathways of the pulp. 10th edition. St Louis (MO): Mosby-Elsevier; 2011. p. 2–39.
86. AAE consensus conference recommended diagnostic terminology. J Endod 2009;35(10):1634.
87. Levin GL, Law AS, Holland GR, et al. Identify and define all diagnostic terms for pulpal health and disease states. J Endod 2009;12:1645–57.
88. Torabinejad M, Shabahang S. Pulp and periapical pathosis. In: Torabinejad M, Walton RE, editors. Principles and practice of endodontics. 4th edition. Philadelphia: WB Saunders; 2009. p. 49–67.
89. American Board of Endodontics. Pulpal and periapical diagnostic terminology. Chicago: American Board of Endodontics; 2007.
90. Glickman GN, Mickel AK, Levin LG, et al. Glossary of endodontic terms. 6th edition. Chicago: American Association of Endodontics; 2003. p. 30, 35, 45.
91. Abbott PV, Yu C. A clinical classification of the status of the pulp and the root canal system. Aust Dent J 2007;52(Suppl):S17–31.
92. Torabinejad M, Eby WC, Nairdorf IJ. Inflammatory and immunological aspects of the pathogenesis of human periapical lesions. J Endod 1985;11:479–88.
93. Marimen D, Green TL, Walton RE, et al. Histologic examination of condensing osteitis. J Endod 1992;18(4):196.

Contemporary Concepts in the Diagnosis of Periodontal Disease

Dana L. Wolf, DMD, MS[a],*, Ira B. Lamster, DDS, MMSc[b]

KEYWORDS

• Periodontal disease • Diagnosis • Probing depth

THE CHALLENGES OF PERIODONTAL DIAGNOSIS

Periodontitis is an inflammatory disease of bacterial origin that results in the progressive destruction of the tissues that support the teeth, specifically the gingiva, periodontal ligament, and alveolar bone. Although there have been significant advances in the understanding of the cause and pathogenesis of periodontal disease over the past 40 years, the traditional methods by which clinicians diagnose periodontal disease have remained virtually unchanged. The diagnosis of periodontal disease relies almost exclusively on clinical parameters and traditional dental radiography. Clinicians use clinical and radiographic findings to diagnose patients according to the classification scheme developed at the 1999 International Workshop for the Classification of Periodontal Diseases and Conditions (**Table 1**). These traditional diagnostic tools have some significant shortcomings. Clinical assessments such as probing depth (PD) and clinical attachment level (CAL) are somewhat subjective and time consuming and therefore underutilized in general dental practice.[1] Studies of the progression of periodontitis have demonstrated that there are periods of active tissue destruction separated by periods of inactive disease;[2–4] however, traditional clinical assessments do not enable a practitioner performing a single routine periodontal examination to determine whether active tissue destruction is occurring. There are, for example, no definitive means of determining whether gingival inflammation in a successfully treated case of periodontitis represents early recurrent disease or gingivitis on a stable but reduced periodontium. Demonstrating progressive loss of periodontal support requires longitudinal assessment. Current diagnostic methodologies do not enable us to accurately predict

a Section of Oral and Diagnostic Sciences, Division of Periodontics, Columbia University College of Dental Medicine, 630 West 168th Street, PH 7E-Room 110, New York, NY 10032, USA
b College of Dental Medicine, Columbia University, 630 West 168th Street, New York, NY 10032, USA
* Corresponding author.
E-mail address: dlw2004@columbia.edu

Dent Clin N Am 55 (2011) 47–61
doi:10.1016/j.cden.2010.08.009
0011-8532/11/$ – see front matter © 2011 Elsevier Inc. All rights reserved.

Table 1
Classification of periodontal diseases and conditions

I. Gingival Diseases	A. Plaque-associated gingival diseases Non–plaque-induced gingival diseases
II. Chronic Periodontitis	B. Localized Generalized
III. Aggressive Periodontitis	C. Localized Generalized
IV. Periodontitis as a Manifestation of Systemic Disease	D. Associated with hematologic disorders Associated with genetic disorders Not otherwise specified
V. Necrotizing Periodontal Diseases	E. Necrotizing ulcerative gingivitis Necrotizing ulcerative periodontitis
VI. Abscesses of the Periodontium	F. Gingival abscess Periodontal abscess Pericoronal abscess
VII. Periodontitis Associated with Endodontic Lesions	G. Combined periodontic-endodontic lesions
VIII. Developmental or Acquired Deformities and Conditions	H. Localized tooth-related factors that modify or predispose Mucogingival deformities and conditions around teeth Mucogingival deformities and conditions on edentulous ridges Occlusal trauma

Adapted from Armitage GC. Development of a classification system for periodontal diseases and conditions. Ann Periodontol 1999;4(1):2, 3; with permission.

which periodontal sites, teeth, or individuals are susceptible to further periodontal breakdown. Given the limitations of current diagnostic tools, researchers are working to develop techniques that address some of these inadequacies. In this article, the authors review the diagnostic techniques currently used and present new approaches and technologies that are being developed to improve the diagnosis of periodontal disease.

CURRENT DIAGNOSTIC STRATEGIES

In response to pathogenic bacteria in dental plaque (a biofilm adherent to the tooth surface), an innate inflammatory response as well as cellular and humoral immune responses are mounted locally in the periodontal tissues. The complex host response is aimed at containing the infectious stimulus and preventing bacterial invasion into the tissues. If the infection cannot be contained, the local release of proinflammatory cytokines and tissue degrading enzymes results in damage to the supporting hard and soft tissues of the tooth. The junctional epithelium becomes ulcerated and migrates apically, and there is destruction of the gingival connective tissue, periodontal ligament, and alveolar bone. Although pathogenic bacteria are capable of degrading host tissues, it is the host's response to pathogenic bacteria rather than the bacteria themselves that is responsible for most of the tissue breakdown associated with periodontitis.[5] The traditional diagnostic methods described in the following sections aim to identify the etiologic factors, assess the clinical signs of the inflammatory process, and determine the degree to which periodontal destruction has occurred.

Assessment of Etiologic Factors

Bacteria are necessary but insufficient by themselves to cause periodontal disease.[6] It is generally accepted that even in the presence of pathogenic bacteria, individuals are variably susceptible to tissue breakdown. Identifying the presence of specific periodontal pathogens in dental plaque is not currently a strategy used to establish a periodontal diagnosis.[1] Nonetheless, because bacteria are the initiating factor (and primary target of most of the present therapeutic modalities), it is important to assess the degree of bacterial plaque present and counsel patients on proper plaque control. It is also important to identify any factor that might make an individual susceptible to the accumulation of dental plaque. Some of these factors include a lack of manual dexterity associated with arthritis or other conditions, a reduced frequency of oral hygiene practices, improper technique, and tooth anatomy that promotes plaque retention.

Susceptibility to periodontitis is conferred by several established risk factors, such as diabetes mellitus and cigarette smoking.[7] Certain genetic syndromes are also associated with periodontal disease.[8] It is for these reasons that a thorough medical history, including a history of cigarette smoking, is an important part of establishing a periodontal diagnosis.

Assessment of Gingival Inflammation

Much information regarding the degree of gingival inflammation can be obtained from a simple visual inspection of the tissues. Healthy gingiva is typically pink and firm and has a knife-edged margin. Inflamed tissues exhibit cardinal signs of inflammation, such as redness and swelling (**Fig. 1**). Bleeding on probing (BOP) is an important indicator of gingival inflammation within the periodontal pocket. It occurs because of microulcerations in the junctional epithelium. BOP is influenced by repeated probe insertions in a short time as well as by the use of excessive force (>25 N). Purulent exudate can also be an important sign of gingival inflammation; however, true suppuration may be difficult to distinguish from plaque that is expressed from the gingival crevice.

Calor, or heat, is another cardinal sign of inflammation and has been investigated as a diagnostic measure of periodontal status. Haffajee and colleagues[9] used a periodontal temperature probe (Periotemp, ABIO-DENT, Inc, Danvers, MA, USA) to

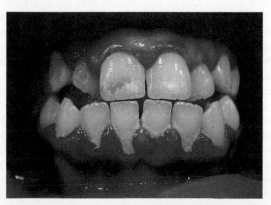

Fig. 1. A patient with plaque-induced gingivitis. There is evidence of the cardinal signs of inflammation, including erythema and edema.

assess subgingival temperature and found that elevated mean subgingival temperature was related to subsequent attachment loss.

Assessment of Loss of Periodontal Attachment

PD assessment is probably the most commonly used clinical measure for detecting loss of periodontal support. It is measured from the free gingival margin (FGM) to the depth of the probable crevice. The depth of a healthy gingival sulcus ranges from 1 to 3 mm. PD is not the most objective measure of loss of periodontal tissues because the position of the FGM is variable. When there is gingival inflammation, the FGM may be located more coronal than normal because of edema in the tissues (the FGM is normally located 1.5–2 mm coronal to the cementoenamel junction [CEJ]). In this situation, there may be a deeper-than-normal PD even in the absence of loss of periodontal attachment. Such a deepened pocket is described as a pseudopocket. A true periodontal pocket occurs when there has been apical migration of the junctional epithelium and loss of supporting tissues of the tooth. The PD may also be normal in the presence of significant attachment loss. This may occur in the case of treated periodontitis or when the disease process manifests with gingival recession rather than pocket formation.

CAL is a more objective measure of loss of periodontal support because it is measured from a fixed point on the tooth, usually the CEJ, if detectable. CAL is defined as the distance between the CEJ and the base of the probable pocket (**Fig. 2**). Because the apical termination of the junctional epithelium is normally located at the CEJ, there should be no CAL when the periodontal tissues are healthy and there is no history of periodontitis. When the gingival margin is located coronal to the CEJ, CAL is measured by subtracting the distance of the FGM to the CEJ from the PD (PD−[FGM−CEJ]). When there is gingival recession, CAL is calculated by adding the PD and the amount of recession. Calculating the CAL can be challenging, and this variable is more often used in research than in everyday clinical practice. Existing CAL also does not give any indication of current disease activity.

When interpreting the PD and CAL measurements made with conventional periodontal probes, it is important to consider that these values depend on the inflammatory state of the tissues. When probing healthy gingival tissues, the periodontal probe generally stops coronal to the apical extent of the junctional epithelium, which is at the CEJ.[10] When the gingiva is inflamed and the gingival connective tissue has been infiltrated by inflammatory cells, there is less resistance to probe penetration and the periodontal probe generally passes apical to the level of the connective tissue attachment.[11,12] As a result, PD and CAL values may be overestimated in inflamed sites and underestimated in healthy sites. The depth of probe penetration may also be influenced by factors such as the diameter of the probe tip, insertion force, and angulation of the probe. Electronic probes were developed to overcome some of these technical difficulties. Electronic probes, such as the Florida probe (Florida Probe Company, Gainesville, FL, USA), have the advantage of controlling insertion force, automatic data capture into a computer, and a higher resolution than manual probes.[13] Electronic probes have the disadvantage of underestimating PD and CAL in untreated patients. Despite some acknowledged problems, manual probes are perfectly acceptable for routine periodontal examinations and provide results comparable to those with electronic probes.[14]

Other clinical variables used to assess the degree of existing periodontal destruction include mobility and the degree of furcation involvement. Tooth mobility may be caused by several factors, but loss of periodontal attachment is one of the more common causes.[15] Both mobility and furcation involvement are important determinants of a tooth's prognosis.

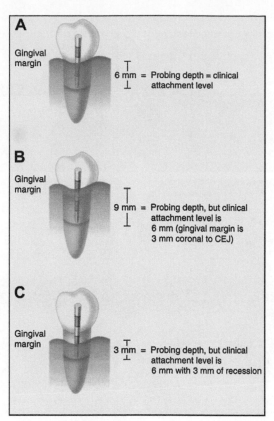

Fig. 2. A depiction of how the parameters PD and CAL relate to one another. (*A*) The gingival margin is at the level of the CEJ, so PD is equal to the CAL. (*B*) The gingival margin is coronal to the CEJ, so the PD is greater than the CAL. (*C*) The PD is within normal limits, but there is gingival recession and significant CAL. (*Adapted from* Armitage, G. Clinical periodontal examination. In: Rose LF, Mealey BL, Genco RJ, et al, editors. Periodontics: medicine, surgery, and implants. St Louis (MO): Elsevier Mosby; 2004. p. 140; with permission.)

RADIOGRAPHIC ASSESSMENT OF PERIODONTAL DISEASE

Radiographs are an essential component of the periodontal examination and indispensable in establishing a periodontal diagnosis. Important information regarding the position and architecture of the alveolar crest of bone is obtained from radiographs. Bite-wings are considered the most accurate intraoral radiographs for determining the height of the alveolar crest. In the absence of bone loss, the alveolar crest is generally located 1 to 2 mm apical to the CEJ (**Fig. 3**A).[16] Vertical bite-wings may need to be taken to visualize the osseous crest in a patient with attachment loss (**Fig. 3**B). Periapical radiographs give the clinician important information regarding crown to root ratio, the periodontal ligament space, and the presence of periapical abnormality. Intraoral radiographs are generally considered preferable to panoramic radiographs for use in periodontal assessment; however, some studies have demonstrated that panoramic radiographs can be used to assess alveolar bone height.[17]

Despite their value in periodontal diagnosis, radiographs have several limitations as diagnostic tools. First, they do not give any information about disease activity or

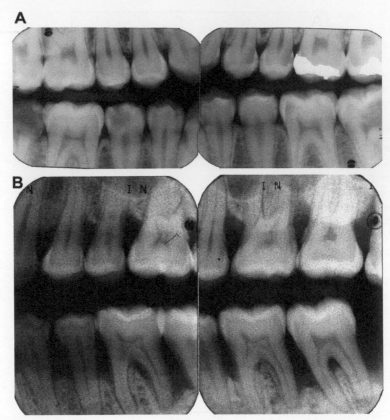

Fig. 3. (A) Horizontal bite-wing radiographs show that the height of the alveolar bone is in a normal position. (B) Vertical bite-wing radiographs demonstrating vertical and horizontal bone loss.

progression. A successfully treated case of periodontitis is likely to have similar pretreatment and posttreatment levels of radiographic bone loss. Second, studies in the periodontal literature have generally demonstrated that radiographs tend to underestimate the amount of attachment loss[18,19] and that clinical changes (attachment loss) precede radiographic changes.[20]

Subtraction radiography is a technique that longitudinally assesses change in bone density. Two radiographs with the same geometry are exposed at 2 different times. The image present in the first film is subtracted from that in the second film. The difference reflects bone gain or loss. The technique can detect bone density changes as low as 5%, whereas sequentially taken conventional radiographs reveal bone changes only after 30% to 50% of the bone has been resorbed.[21] Subtraction radiography has evolved with the introduction of intraoral digital radiography, and some of the shortcomings of the original technique have been addressed.[22] Nonetheless, this technique is generally not used in clinical practice.

SUPPLEMENTAL DIAGNOSTIC TESTS

The clinical and radiographic assessments described earlier are the most commonly used measures of periodontal disease. However, there are several supplemental tests that have been developed to address the fact that traditional approaches do not adequately identify patients or sites with progressive disease (or at risk for progressive disease). Supplemental tests may also be used to assess the response to therapy and determine appropriate recall intervals.[23] For several reasons, these tests, which include microbial, biochemical, and genetic tests, are not routinely used in clinical practice. However, many of these tests offer the clinician information that is not available from current diagnostic procedures.

Microbial Testing

Although there are different bacterial species associated with gingival health and disease, microbial testing is not currently used to establish a periodontal diagnosis. Whether the presence of certain bacteria may help distinguish between different forms of periodontitis (chronic vs aggressive) is currently a matter of controversy.[24] In a systematic review, Mombelli and colleagues[25] found that the presence or absence of certain identified periodontal pathogens could not distinguish cases of chronic periodontitis from cases of aggressive periodontitis. Other possible uses of microbial testing are for selection of an appropriate systemic antibiotic, assessment of therapeutic outcomes, and/or risk assessment. There are several methods for detecting bacteria in dental plaque. These include bacterial culture, immunologic assays, enzymatic assays, and molecular biologic techniques that detect bacterial DNA or RNA.

Bacterial culture is the gold standard against which new microbial tests are compared. It involves growing bacteria in either aerobic or anaerobic conditions on different media and performing tests to identify and quantify specific species. This technique enables the characterization of pathogens as well as the determination of antibiotic susceptibility. The drawbacks of culture are that the plaque sample must contain viable bacteria and that some putative pathogens are difficult to cultivate.[24]

Immunologic methods use antibodies that target specific bacterial antigens. When the antibodies bind their antigen, the reaction can be visualized by techniques such as direct and indirect immunofluorescent microscopic assays, flow cytometry, and enzyme-linked immunosorbent assay.[24] Immunologic techniques enable the identification and quantification (or semiquantification) of bacteria. However, the only bacteria that are identified are those for which specific antibodies are available.

Several putative periodontal pathogens such as *Porphyromonas gingivalis*, *Tannerella forsythia*, and *Aggregatibacter actinomycetemcomitans* possess in common a trypsinlike enzyme that hydrolyzes a substrate *N*-benzoyl-DL-arginine-2-naphthylamide (BANA). A diagnostic test that measures the activity of this trypsinlike enzyme was developed so as to identify the presence of oral bacteria that produce the enzyme. Loesche and colleagues[26] published a study comparing the BANA test to other methods of microbial testing and found that the BANA test had similar sensitivity as the other techniques that were evaluated. The BANA test is easy to perform chairside and was commercially available for a brief period in the 1990s. Serious limitations of the test include its inability to distinguish between individual bacteria, the ability to detect pathogens only when they are present in high numbers, and the fact that its diagnostic utility has not been validated in clinical trials.[24]

Molecular biologic techniques use the bacterial genome as a means of identifying specific bacteria. DNA isolated and purified from plaque samples can be analyzed via nucleic acid probes or polymerase chain reaction (PCR). Nucleic acid probes are synthesized sequences of DNA or RNA that are complementary to specific nucleic acid sequences in the bacterial genome. Bacteria can be identified when DNA isolated from dental plaque is hybridized (paired with complementary DNA) with species-specific probes that are labeled to allow visualization.[24] Checkerboard hybridization is a technique that uses probes to simultaneously test for the presence of up to 43 bacterial species.[27] Checkerboard hybridization enables rapid processing of numerous plaque samples and is often used for research purposes. PCR uses a DNA replicating enzyme (polymerase) to amplify target sequences of DNA. Standard PCR is not a quantitative assessment of identified bacteria, although a technique called real-time PCR does enable quantification. Tests that use the genome have the advantage of not requiring viable bacteria, but they are costly and require sophisticated laboratory equipment, so they are not practical for routine clinical use.[24]

Biochemical Analysis as Part of Periodontal Diagnosis

The biochemical assessment of periodontal disease can be accomplished using several approaches. The most practical and least-invasive approach involves analysis of biologic fluids that are derived from the periodontal tissues or contain specific mediators that are present as a result of periodontal disease. The biologic fluids that have been studied to understand the nature of destructive periodontitis and to identify potential diagnostic markers of active disease include serum (blood), gingival fluid, and saliva.

As the understanding of the pathophysiology of periodontal disease advanced in the 1970s, researchers began to analyze serum to identify the nature of the host's response in periodontal disease.[28,29] Studies of serum antibody levels to periodontal bacteria were among the earliest investigations demonstrating that a humoral immune response occurs in patients with periodontitis. More recent studies have demonstrated that patients with periodontitis have elevated antibody titers to subgingival pathogens.[30] Recently, serum levels of markers of the inflammatory response have been studied for their relationship to periodontitis. The levels of inflammatory cytokines (ie, interleukin [IL]-6) and general markers of inflammation (ie, C-reactive protein) have been shown to be elevated in the blood of patients with periodontitis.[31] Nevertheless, serum markers of periodontititis, or of inflammation, are not currently used as diagnostic tests for periodontitis.

Gingival crevicular fluid (GCF) is a serum transudate, or more commonly an inflammatory exudate, that emanates from the gingival crevice and can be collected from the orifice of the crevice. A great deal of attention has been placed on the analysis of GCF for diagnostic purposes. GCF collection is most commonly accomplished with the use of small methylcellulose filter paper strips placed within the crevice or at the orifice. There has been a debate regarding the technical aspects of collecting GCF and reporting the data (as concentration or total amount of mediator in a timed collection). The reasons for this debate include the variable amount of fluid that can be collected at different tooth sites and the observation that the collection procedure can influence fluid volume, because the insertion of a filter strip can, over time, cause disruption of the underlying capillary bed. At present, most studies use a timed (30 seconds) insertion of the GCF strip to the depth of the sulcus or pocket. This procedure eliminates the need for the determination of the volume of fluid that was collected (this volume can be determined using an electronic meter known as the Periotron [Oraflow Inc, Smithtown, NY, USA])[32] and allows for the comparison of samples based on the standardized collection time.

A wide variety of mediators have been studied in GCF.[33] These mediators can generally be classified as assessing the host immune or inflammatory response or metabolic markers associated with periodontitis. The former includes antibodies, proteases and other enzymes (including the matrix metalloproteinases [MMPs]), proinflammatory cytokines (ie, IL-1β, IL-6, IL-17, tumor necrosis factor [TNF]-α), and other molecules in the different inflammatory cascades (ie, prostaglandin E$_2$). Measures of tissue metabolism include markers of cell necrosis (ie, the enzymes lactate dehydrogenase and aspartate transaminase), molecules that play a role in the response to oxidative stress (ie, glutathione), growth factors (ie, transforming growth factor β), and measures of bone remodeling and turnover (ie, receptor activated nuclear factor-κB ligand [RANKL] and osteoprotegerin). At present, markers of inflammation have received the most attention. Several of these markers have been evaluated for their relationship to active, progressive periodontitis in clinical trials, and 2 diagnostic tests based on the analysis of elastase and aspartate aminotransferase were available commercially as chair-side tests for the diagnosis of periodontitis.

GCF has also been analyzed with infrared (IR) spectroscopy. IR spectroscopy is a technique that involves the analysis of biologic fluids to quantitatively determine analytes of interest.[34] Vibrating covalent bonds of organic molecules absorb a characteristic wavelength of IR light. The spectrum of absorbed light may be used to establish a molecular fingerprint of a tissue or fluid.[35] IR analysis of GCF has recently been shown to distinguish between periodontal health and disease.[36] Longitudinal studies are needed to determine whether IR can be used to predict the risk for progressive disease.

Despite the enormous interest in the biochemical analysis of GCF, the use of this fluid as the basis of a diagnostic test has not been embraced by the profession. The reasons relate to difficulty in developing a logical and practical strategy for sampling GCF. The filter paper strips collect fluid only from a 2- to 3-mm wide portion of the crevice. To assess the entire dentition, sampling of GCF has traditionally occurred at a preestablished site on each tooth (ie, the mesiobuccal line angle of each tooth). This procedure is time consuming and may not capture a sample that is representative of the entire periodontium.

A more practical approach to the biochemical diagnosis of periodontal disease is offered by the analysis of saliva. Saliva has been analyzed as a diagnostic fluid in medicine,[37] and the analysis of saliva also offers intriguing possibilities as the basis of diagnostic tests for oral disease. Whole saliva can be collected noninvasively and analyzed for the presence of markers that, in general, are derived from GCF and have been shown to be associated with the risk for active periodontal destruction. The markers include enzymes that indicate cell necrosis and tissue destruction and inflammatory markers, such as TNF-α, IL-1β, MMP-8, and the neutrophil-derived enzyme, β-glucuronidase. Studies have shown these markers to be elevated in the saliva of patients with periodontitis.[38]

As technologies evolve, saliva may also be analyzed for genomic and microbial markers of periodontal disease.[39] Salivary RNA has been identified and used in the diagnosis of oral cancer and Sjögren syndrome; however, to date there are no salivary DNA or RNA biomarkers for periodontal disease.[39] The National Institute of Dental and Craniofacial Research has recognized the potential in salivary diagnostics and is funding research that uses microfluidic and microelectromechanical systems for point-of-care testing for oral disease. These systems use small sample and reagent volumes to detect and measure proteins, DNA, RNA, bacteria, electrolytes, and other molecules in saliva. Researchers are developing lab-on-a-chip devices that will enable rapid and simultaneous detection of multiple biomarkers. Herr and colleagues[40] have been working on developing a portable device that can measure multiple biomarkers and are looking to characterize groups of proteins that are associated with different stages of periodontal disease.

As the detection of biomarkers in saliva improves, this biologic fluid may become an important part of periodontal diagnosis. Saliva-based diagnostic tests do not give tooth- or site-specific information, rather they give patient measures that may be used in several ways. A salivary test may be used as a home screening tool that is based on a color change or simple color scale. A positive test result would indicate the need for a comprehensive dental evaluation. Alternatively, a salivary diagnostic test can be used as a quantitative in-office test that is used as part of the initial patient evaluation to assess the effectiveness of treatment and to monitor patient status during regular recall visits.

Genetic Testing

Although it is generally accepted that there is a genetic susceptibility to periodontitis,[41,42] the genes that confer susceptibility have not been definitively established. Several candidate genes have been proposed as putative risk or prognostic factors. In 1997, Kornman and colleagues[43] published a landmark study that found polymorphisms (interindividual differences in DNA sequences coding for 1 specific gene, giving rise to different functional and/or morphologic traits) in the gene for IL-1 to be a severity factor for periodontitis. A diagnostic test based on the carriage of the IL-1 polymorphism was developed and is commercially available. The test has not been widely adopted because it is of questionable clinical utility and it is unclear whether available data support its use. Since the publication of the Kornman study, polymorphisms in several genes have been proposed as risk markers for periodontitis.[44–46]

Overall, the literature on the role of individual polymorphisms is conflicting and difficult to interpret. Because periodontitis is a complex disease, it is likely that multiple genes contribute to disease susceptibility. A more comprehensive approach to the search for candidate genes should be considered. For example, Brett and colleagues[47] investigated multiple polymorphisms and their carriage among subjects with chronic and aggressive periodontitis. A relatively new method of genetic analysis, microarray technology, enables the analysis of thousands of genes at once. Using microarrays, investigators can examine which genes are differentially expressed in periodontitis. Demmer and colleagues[48] extracted messenger RNA from healthy and diseased gingival tissue and used microarrays to assess gene expression. Genes involved in apoptosis, antigen presentation, and antimicrobial humoral response were among those differentially expressed among diseased and healthy tissues. Microarray technology is a valuable tool for insight into the genetic susceptibility and pathobiology of periodontitis. As technologies evolve, it is easy to imagine the availability of a chair-side test for genetic susceptibility to periodontitis.

Newly Emerging Noninvasive Methods for Periodontal Diagnosis

Near infrared (NIR) spectroscopy is a test that provides a measure of oxygen saturation of the tissues.[35] Liu and colleagues[49] assessed multiple indices of periodontal inflammation using NIR spectroscopy and found that the tissue oxygenation at periodontitis sites was significantly decreased compared with that in patients with gingivitis and healthy controls. The investigators postulated that the tissue hypoxia reflects increased oxygen consumption that occurs with persistent inflammation. This finding is consistent with the fact that putative periodontal pathogens are generally anaerobic. NIR spectroscopy of the periodontal tissues was performed using a special intraoral probe.

Other noninvasive methods that have been suggested for imaging of the periodontal tissues include optical coherence tomography (OCT), acoustic microstreaming (ultrasonography), and cone beam computed tomography (CBCT). OCT creates high-resolution, cross-sectional images using a focused light beam that is scanned across the tissues of interest. Preliminary data have demonstrated that OCT could provide high-resolution, 3-dimensional imaging of periodontal soft and hard tissues.[35] Although some researchers have considered ultrasonography as an imaging tool for the perio-dontium,[50,51] use of this technology for periodontal diagnosis is not developed.

Computed tomography (CT) enables cross-sectional, 3-dimensional analysis of mineralized tissue without distortion. CT scans are potentially informative for peri-odontal diagnosis; however, they are not used for this purpose because of the high cost of the machine, high levels of radiation, and relatively low resolution.[52] CBCT scan-ners on the other hand are much cheaper and impart much less radiation to the patient. Misch and colleagues[52] compared the accuracy of CBCT, periapical radiography, and direct measurement with a periodontal probe in measuring artificially created osseous defect in mandibles of dry skulls. Misch and colleagues suggested that CBCT has advantages over radiographs because it enables visualization of defects in 3 dimen-sions and visualization of buccal and lingual defects. A more recent in vitro study simi-larly reported better diagnostic and quantitative information on periodontal bone levels from CBCT compared with conventional radiography.[53] Additional research is indi-cated to determine the feasibility of using CBCT in the assessment of periodontitis.

SUMMARY

For all health care disciplines, clinical signs and symptoms play a critical role in estab-lishing a diagnosis. Diagnostic tests are used adjunctively to provide information that is not available from clinical findings. Such tests include microscopic evaluation of tissue (biopsy), evaluation of bodily fluids for markers of disease, imaging studies, and identification of specific microbial pathogens. Genetic analysis is also becoming an important area of study as the genetic contribution to specific diseases is elucidated.

The addition of a diagnostic test to patient evaluation is meaningful only if the test provides additional diagnostic information over what is obtained from the clinical assessment or if it helps guide the treatment more effectively. At present, diagnostic tests that aid in the assessment and management of patients with periodontitis are not a routine part of dental practice. Historically, this is likely because of the accessibility of the oral cavity to clinical and radiographic examination. Nevertheless, it has become clear that clinical and radiographic assessments fail to provide important information regarding the patient's disease, including whether there is the risk for transition from gingivitis to periodontitis, the disease is in a quiescent or destructive phase, adequate treatment has been provided, or there is the risk for disease recurrence. Development of a diagnostic test with appropriate sensitivity and specificity that provides this infor-mation would be invaluable in the management of patients with periodontal disease (**Fig. 4**).

One innovative approach to diagnosis and risk assessment for periodontal disease is the PreVisor software program (Previser Corporation, Mount Vernon, WA, USA), which is a risk assessment tool for patients with periodontal disease. Based on the longitudinal data that followed the progression of periodontal disease over a 15-year period, an algorithm that allows patients to be assessed for risk for periodontal destruction and tooth loss was developed.[54] The clinician enters specific information about each patient, including a history of dental care, smoking history, presence of diabetes mellitus, and existing dental or periodontal findings. These data are used to calculate the severity of disease and the risk for future disease progression. The disease state is expressed on a 0 to 100 scale, and a risk score is expressed on a 1 to 5 scale, with 1 as very low risk and 5 as very high risk. The severity of the patient's periodontitis and the risk score can be plotted against time (**Fig. 5**). Thus far, the advantages of using this risk assessment tool have not been fully explored.

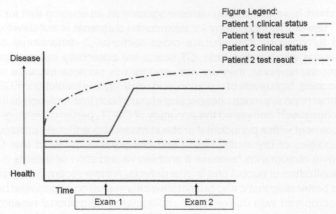

Figure Legend:
Patient 1 clinical status ——
Patient 1 test result — · —
Patient 2 clinical status ———
Patient 2 test result — · · —

Fig. 4. The ideal diagnostic test would be able to predict the development of disease before clinical signs and symptoms. At the first examination, patients 1 (*green*) and 2 (*red*) have similar levels of disease; however, the test results are different. At the second examination, the level of disease of patient 1 has remained the same, whereas that of patient 2 has worsened. The test result remains elevated for patient 2.

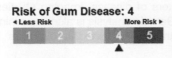

Risk of Gum Disease: 4
◄ Less Risk   More Risk ►

Risk predicts your future disease state. Your risk is determined by risk factor which are distinct from the signs and symptoms of disease. Preventing disea requires treatment that reduces your risk factors. With routine dental care, to loss is 10 times more likely for an individual who has very high (5) risk compared to an individual who has low (2) risk. However, when risk is used to guide the selection of special treatment, tooth loss can be reduced 50% to 100%.
Your risk score of 4 is reflected against the chart to the left.

Disease State 13
Localized mild and moderate periodontitis
Your disease state reflects the amount of damage caused by gum disease. As the disease state worsens, treatment increases in amount, complexity and cost. Tooth loss and the failure rate of repairs are greater for individuals with higher disease state score Treatment can repair the damage caused by disease, but tends not to help much in preventing new disease. Disease prevention requires treatment that reduces your risk factors. The best treatment incorporates both repair (where needed) and prevention.

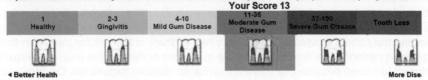

Your Score 13

◄ Better Health   More Dise

What Changed The information below shows the progression of your risk scores:

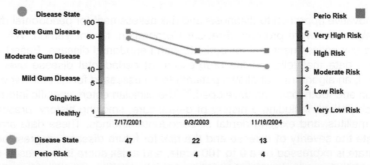

	7/17/2001	9/3/2003	11/16/2004
Disease State	47	22	13
Perio Risk	5	4	4

Fig. 5. Sample report from Previser.com. (Available at: http://www.previser.com/documents/reports/f39000c7-81a1-45fd-bb1f-f45d99245dbe_pf.html. Accessed May 26, 2010; with permission.)

With the enormous focus on the potential impact of periodontal disease and oral inflammation on diseases and disorders at distant sites, a diagnostic test based on the presence of important inflammatory mediators may offer a quantitative measure of the oral inflammatory burden. Such a test would help guide the clinician concerned with the effect of periodontal inflammation on morbidity associated with cardiovascular or cerebrovascular disease, adverse obstetric outcomes, diabetes mellitus, and other disorders. The test could be used to assess whether periodontal therapy has successfully reduced this risk.

New approaches to periodontal diagnosis, including biochemical tests and the application of devices that assess the periodontal tissues, have been shown to provide the clinician with information not available by traditional means. The widespread application of these tests will depend on several factors, including ease of use, cost, the strength of the data supporting the value of the tests, and the ability of the test to aid in patient management. Use of validated diagnostic tests for periodontal disease will also require a paradigm shift in the approach of the dental profession to disease management. Dentists will spend more time on the diagnostic phase of treatment, and the result will be better treatment outcomes.

REFERENCES

1. Chapple IL. Periodontal diagnosis and treatment; where does the future lie? Periodontol 2000 2009;51(1):9–24.
2. Goodson JM, Tanner AC, Haffajee AD, et al. Patterns of progression and regression of advanced destructive periodontal disease. J Clin Periodontol 1982;9(6): 472–81.
3. Haffajee AD, Socransky SS, Goodson JM. Periodontal disease activity. J Periodont Res 1982;17(5):521–2.
4. Socransky SS, Haffajee AD, Goodson JM, et al. New concepts of destructive periodontal disease. J Clin Periodontol 1984;11(1):21–32.
5. Offenbacher S. Periodontal diseases: pathogenesis. Ann Periodontol 1996;1(1): 821–78.
6. Page RC. Critical issues in periodontal research. J Dent Res 1995;74(4):1118–28.
7. Papapanou PN. Periodontal diseases: epidemiology. Ann Periodontol 1996;1(1): 1–36.
8. Kinane DF, Shiba H, Hart TC. The genetic basis of periodontitis. Periodontol 2000. 2005;39:91–117.
9. Haffajee AD, Socransky SS, Goodson JM. Subgingival temperature (II). Relation to future periodontal attachment loss. J Clin Periodontol 1992;19(6):409–16.
10. Listgarten MA, Mao R, Robinson PJ. Periodontal probing and the relationship of the probe tip to periodontal tissues. J Periodontol 1976;47(9):511–3.
11. Robinson PJ, Vitek RM. The relationship between gingival inflammation and resistance to probe penetration. J Periodont Res 1979;14(3):239–43.
12. Fowler C, Garrett S, Crigger M, et al. Histologic probe position in treated and untreated human periodontal tissues. J Clin Periodontol 1982;9(5):373–85.
13. Reddy MS. The use of periodontal probes and radiographs in clinical trials of diagnostic tests. Ann Periodontol 1997;2(1):113–22.
14. Greenstein G. Contemporary interpretation of probing depth assessments: diagnostic and therapeutic implications. A literature review. J Periodontol 1997; 68(12):1194–205.
15. Muhlemann HR. Tooth mobility: a review of clinical aspects and research findings. J Periodontol 1967;38(6):686–713.

16. Hausmann E, Allen K, Clerehugh V. What alveolar crest level on a bite-wing radiograph represents bone loss? J Periodontol 1991;62(9):570–2.
17. Walsh TF, al-Hokail OS, Fosam EB. The relationship of bone loss observed on panoramic radiographs with clinical periodontal screening. J Clin Periodontol 1997;24(3):153–7.
18. Suomi JD, Plumbo J, Barbano JP. A comparative study of radiographs and pocket measurements in periodontal disease evaluation. J Periodontol 1968; 39(6):311–5.
19. Akesson L, Hakansson J, Rohlin M. Comparison of panoramic and intraoral radiography and pocket probing for the measurement of the marginal bone level. J Clin Periodontol 1992;19(5):326–32.
20. Goodson JM, Haffajee AD, Socransky SS. The relationship between attachment level loss and alveolar bone loss. J Clin Periodontol 1984;11(5):348–59.
21. Jeffcoat MK, Reddy MS. A comparison of probing and radiographic methods for detection of periodontal disease progression. Curr Opin Dent 1991;1(1):45–51.
22. Reddy MS, Jeffcoat MK. Digital subtraction radiography. Dent Clin North Am 1993;37(4):553–65.
23. Armitage GC. Diagnosis of periodontal diseases. J Periodontol 2003;74(8): 1237–47.
24. Sanz M, Lau L, Herrera D, et al. Methods of detection of Actinobacillus actinomycetemcomitans, Porphyromonas gingivalis and Tannerella forsythensis in periodontal microbiology, with special emphasis on advanced molecular techniques: a review. J Clin Periodontol 2004;31(12):1034–47.
25. Mombelli A, Casagni F, Madianos PN. Can presence or absence of periodontal pathogens distinguish between subjects with chronic and aggressive periodontitis? A systematic review. J Clin Periodontol 2002;29(Suppl 3):10–21 [discussion: 37–18].
26. Loesche WJ, Lopatin DE, Giordano J, et al. Comparison of the benzoyl-DL-arginine-naphthylamide (BANA) test, DNA probes, and immunological reagents for ability to detect anaerobic periodontal infections due to Porphyromonas gingivalis, Treponema denticola, and Bacteroides forsythus. J Clin Microbiol 1992;30(2): 427–33.
27. Socransky SS, Smith C, Martin L, et al. "Checkerboard" DNA-DNA hybridization. Biotechniques 1994;17(4):788–92.
28. Ebersole JL, Taubman MA, Smith DJ, et al. Human immune responses to oral microorganisms. II. Serum antibody responses to antigens from Actinobacillus actinomycetemcomitans and the correlation with localized juvenile periodontitis. J Clin Immunol 1983;3(4):321–31.
29. Ebersole JL, Taubman MA, Smith DJ, et al. Humoral immune responses and diagnosis of human periodontal disease. J Periodont Res 1982;17(5):478–80.
30. Papapanou PN, Neiderud AM, Disick E, et al. Longitudinal stability of serum immunoglobulin G responses to periodontal bacteria. J Clin Periodontol 2004; 31(11):985–90.
31. Loos BG, Craandijk J, Hoek FJ, et al. Elevation of systemic markers related to cardiovascular diseases in the peripheral blood of periodontitis patients. J Periodontol 2000;71(10):1528–34.
32. Bul P, Dreyer WP, Grobler SR. The periotron gingival crevicular fluid meter. J Periodont Res 1986;21(1):39–44.
33. Loos BG, Tjoa S. Host-derived diagnostic markers for periodontitis: do they exist in gingival crevice fluid? Periodontol 2000. 2005;39:53–72.
34. Jackson M, Sowa MG, Mantsch HH. Infrared spectroscopy: a new frontier in medicine. Biophys Chem 1997;68(1–3):109–25.

35. Xiang X, Sowa MG, Iacopino AM, et al. An update on novel non-invasive approaches for periodontal diagnosis. J Periodontol 2010;81(2):186–98.
36. Xiang XM, Liu KZ, Man A, et al. Periodontitis-specific molecular signatures in gingival crevicular fluid. J Periodont Res 2010;45(3):345–52.
37. Mandel ID. The diagnostic uses of saliva. J Oral Pathol Med 1990;19(3):119–25.
38. Lamster IB, Ahlo JK. Analysis of gingival crevicular fluid as applied to the diagnosis of oral and systemic diseases. Ann N Y Acad Sci 2007;1098:216–29.
39. Zhang L, Henson BS, Camargo PM, et al. The clinical value of salivary biomarkers for periodontal disease. Periodontol 2000. 2009;51:25–37.
40. Herr AE, Hatch AV, Giannobile WV, et al. Integrated microfluidic platform for oral diagnostics. Ann N Y Acad Sci 2007;1098:362–74.
41. Michalowicz BS, Aeppli D, Virag JG, et al. Periodontal findings in adult twins. J Periodontol 1991;62(5):293–9.
42. de Heens GL, Loos BG, van der Velden U. Monozygotic twins are discordant for chronic periodontitis: clinical and bacteriological findings. J Clin Periodontol 2010;37(2):120–8.
43. Kornman KS, Crane A, Wang HY, et al. The interleukin-1 genotype as a severity factor in adult periodontal disease. J Clin Periodontol 1997;24(1):72–7.
44. Kobayashi T, Sugita N, van der Pol WL, et al. The Fc gamma receptor genotype as a risk factor for generalized early-onset periodontitis in Japanese patients. J Periodontol 2000;71(9):1425–32.
45. de Souza AP, Trevilatto PC, Scarel-Caminaga RM, et al. MMP-1 promoter polymorphism: association with chronic periodontitis severity in a Brazilian population. J Clin Periodontol 2003;30(2):154–8.
46. Craandijk J, van Krugten MV, Verweij CL, et al. Tumor necrosis factor-alpha gene polymorphisms in relation to periodontitis. J Clin Periodontol 2002;29(1):28–34.
47. Brett PM, Zygogianni P, Griffiths GS, et al. Functional gene polymorphisms in aggressive and chronic periodontitis. J Dent Res 2005;84(12):1149–53.
48. Demmer RT, Behle JH, Wolf DL, et al. Transcriptomes in healthy and diseased gingival tissues. J Periodontol 2008;79(11):2112–24.
49. Liu KZ, Xiang XM, Man A, et al. In vivo determination of multiple indices of periodontal inflammation by optical spectroscopy. J Periodont Res 2009;44(1):117–24.
50. Spranger H. Ultra-sonic diagnosis of marginal periodontal diseases. Int Dent J 1971;21(4):442–55.
51. Palou ME, McQuade MJ, Rossmann JA. The use of ultrasound for the determination of periodontal bone morphology. J Periodontol 1987;58(4):262–5.
52. Misch KA, Yi ES, Sarment DP. Accuracy of cone beam computed tomography for periodontal defect measurements. J Periodontol 2006;77(7):1261–6.
53. Mol A, Balasundaram A. In vitro cone beam computed tomography imaging of periodontal bone. Dentomaxillofac Radiol 2008;37(6):319–24.
54. Page RC, Krall EA, Martin J, et al. Validity and accuracy of a risk calculator in predicting periodontal disease. J Am Dent Assoc 2002;133(5):569–76.

Contemporary Concepts in the Diagnosis of Oral Cancer and Precancer

Easwar Natarajan, BDS, DMSc[a],*, Ellen Eisenberg, DMD[a,b]

KEYWORDS

- Oral cancer • Squamous cell carcinoma • Leukoplakia
- Precancer • Epithelial dysplasia

Oral cancer is a diagnosis that patients fear and every oral health care provider dreads having to convey. In daily practice of dentistry and medicine, most pathologic conditions are reactive, inflammatory, and perhaps infectious in nature. Malignant neoplasms, including oral cancer (ie, squamous cell carcinoma [SCC]), occur infrequently. Why then, is the fear of oral cancer so pervasive and intense? Almost certainly, it is because both the disease and its treatment conjure a unique spectrum of images associated with profound morbidity. Mental portraits of disfigurement, unrelenting function loss, protracted pain, and even death decrease within the cascade of associations triggered by a diagnosis of oral cancer. Risk for recurrent disease, distant metastases, and susceptibility for developing second primary carcinomas of the upper aerodigestive tract as a product of field cancerization are among the biologic specters linked to a diagnosis of oral cancer.

Despite important advances in the approach to treatment of oral cancer, 5-year survival from the time of diagnosis has remained disappointingly static over the past 50 years. What accounts for this dismal prognosis? The answer to that question is multifaceted, but the poor outlook is in part attributable to late-stage diagnoses with advanced disease. In more than 50% of cases of oral cancer, tumors have already spread distantly before being diagnosed. This situation suggests that many providers, or their patients, or both, are either failing to recognize early oral mucosal changes that indicate cancer development or they are evading timely clinical evaluation of such findings. In stark contrast, in cases in which a primary tumor is localized

[a] Section of Oral and Maxillofacial Pathology, University of Connecticut Health Center, 263 Farmington Avenue MC-0925, Farmington, CT 06030-0925, USA
[b] UConn Oral Pathology Biopsy Service, University of Connecticut Health Center, 263 Farmington Avenue MC-0925, Farmington, CT 06030-0925, USA
* Corresponding author.
E-mail address: natarajan@uchc.edu

Dent Clin N Am 55 (2011) 63–88
doi:10.1016/j.cden.2010.08.006
0011-8532/11/$ – see front matter © 2011 Elsevier Inc. All rights reserved.

dental.theclinics.com

and there is no evidence of metastasis to locoregional lymph nodes at diagnosis, the outlook for survival at 5 years is significantly better. What does this tell us? That the earlier an oral cancer is diagnosed, the better the prospects for improved survival. Given the ready anatomic accessibility of the oral cavity for visual and tactile examination, detecting potentially malignant (ie, precancerous, preinvasive) oral mucosal lesions before they have attained even incipient malignant status should not be insurmountable.

How can clinicians best position themselves to diagnose oral cancer at an early clinical stage of the disease? They must be informed. Contemporary clinicians must have an understanding of the pathogenesis of a disease in which oral surface epithelium that is presumably normal at outset transforms to a malignant state over an extended period. Such understanding must include awareness of the environmental influences, internal and external, that are associated with this transformation, and that are instrumental for identifying individuals at greatest risk for developing the disease. Informed clinicians are best prepared to recognize the spectrum of clinical findings that are most suspicious for evolving (ie, premalignant) or incipient oral cancer lesions. They know the most appropriate approach to take when a suspect oral lesion has been discovered, because that ensures that an accurate diagnosis is obtained expeditiously. They are aware of the long-term implications of a diagnosis of oral precancer or cancer, so that a reasonable and realistic plan for proper clinical follow-up is instituted.

Several issues are addressed in our discussion of contemporary concepts in the approach to diagnosis of oral cancer. We should clarify the term oral cancer. The literature is replete with statistics concerning oral cancer referable to a single broadly diverse anatomic region that encompasses the lips, the oral cavity proper, and the tonsils, oropharynx, and larynx. The problem with combining these various sites into a single location is that there is mounting evidence to suggest that the SCCs that arise in each of these respective regions are associated with different risk factors, morbidities, and progressions toward mortality. Therefore, much of our discussion of oral cancer epidemiology and diagnosis is confined to SCCs of the oral cavity proper, that is, the anatomic region that extends from the mucosa of the lips anteriorly, to the anterior tonsillar pillars and the oral portion of the tongue, posteriorly. Key aspects of the biologic basis of oral cancer development, and the known risk factors associated with the disease are summarized. The clinical presentation of oral cancers and precancerous lesions, and their histopathologic correlates, is discussed. The importance of conventional tissue biopsy as the prevailing gold standard for diagnosis is emphasized. Other current technologies available for detecting and diagnosing oral cancer and premalignant lesions are acknowledged, and their respective strengths and weaknesses are discussed.

EPIDEMIOLOGY

Of 1.5 million cancers diagnosed in the United States annually, oral cancer (SCC) accounts for less than 3% of all cases.[1-3] Globally, it is the sixth most common cancer.[1] The incidence is especially high in the Indian subcontinent, Brazil, Sub-Saharan Africa, Australia and other regions. Oral SCC is the most common malignancy in Southeast Asia.

Incidence of Oral SCC

In a review of statistics, the SEER (Surveillance Epidemiology and End Results) data estimated that 35,720 individuals (25,240 men and 10,480 women) would be diagnosed with cancer of the oral cavity and pharynx in 2009, and that 7600 men and women in the United States would die of the disease.[1] Reading these estimates, the epidemiologic factors and pathogenetic mechanisms that contribute to oral cavity, pharyngeal, and laryngeal SCCs, respectively are similar, but not identical. However, cancer-related data from these sites are often presented collectively. This strategy has resulted in the mistaken implication that the data pertain to a single disease entity. Similarly, several studies also include data from lip cancers in their discussions of oral cancer. However, the cause of cancer of the external lip differs considerably from that of cancer of the oral cavity, and the pharynx and larynx. Therefore, lip cancer data should be considered separately.

It is important to define the anatomic boundaries of the oral cavity to better understand the unique incidence, pathogenetic factors, and consequences of oral SCC. The oral cavity begins anteriorly at the vermilion-mucosal junction of the lips and extends posteriorly to include the base of the oral tongue and the anterior tonsillar pillars. It does not include the pharynx and larynx. Separated in this manner, SCCs of the oral cavity proper (ie, excluding the tonsils, pharynx, larynx, and vermilion-skin portions of the lips) account for approximately 17,000 new cancer cases annually and result in an estimated 6000 deaths per year.[1]

Age, Race, and Sex

It has been long recognized that oral SCC, like many other neoplasms, is a disease of age (**Fig. 1**). In 2009, the median age at diagnosis for SCC of the oral cavity was 61 years.[1] The increased incidence of oral SCCs with age is consistent with the current understanding that, like most malignant neoplasms, oral cancer results from mutations accumulated over a long period. These mutations result in irreversible multifaceted deregulation of cellular homeostasis and eventuate in aberrant differentiation, growth, and replication that, in turn, affect genetic stability, cell aging, apoptosis, carcinogen-mediated mutagenesis, and immune surveillance.[4,5]

In recent decades the incidence rate for oral SCC in men has steadily declined, whereas in women it has remained stable. This finding translates into a relative increase in incidence of oral SCC in women. From 1975 to 2006, both black and white women had similar incidence rates of oral SCC; however, black men have consistently had a 30% higher rate than white men. Similar findings have been reported relative to associated mortality in African American men with oral SCC: the rates remained generally stable or increased between 1975 and 2006. Asian and Hispanic people manifest the lowest rates of oral SCC in the United States.[1]

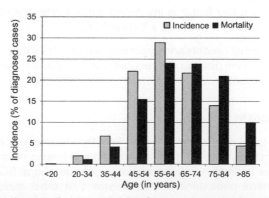

Fig. 1. Oral SCC is a disease of age. Incidence of SCC and resulting mortality in the United States, 2002 to 2006 (SEER).

Site-specific Epidemiology

In the United States, SCC of the oral tongue is the most commonly reported site (36.2% of all oral SCC), followed closely by the floor of the mouth (24.5%).[6,7] As discussed in the section on clinical features, the lateral tongue and the floor of the mouth comprise more than 60% of the so-called cancer-prone locations in the oral cavity.[8,9] Other locations that figure prominently in the SEER data are the tonsillar pillars and retromolar pad areas (20%), followed by the soft palate, lower labial mucosa, buccal mucosa, and gingiva ($\sim$19%). In the United States the buccal mucosa is the sixth most common oral cancer site. Only gingival carcinomas are less common. In striking contrast, the buccal mucosa is the most common location for oral SCC in some other parts of the world (Central and Southeast Asia). The differences in site-specific incidence are likely attributable to cultural differences in the way tobacco and related products are used relative to their mode of delivery (smoking vs chewing). Direct mucosal contact with smokeless tobacco and other noncombustible preparations (eg, paan/betel nut/gutka) seems to account for the predominance of buccal and gingival carcinomas in the non-US oral SCC cases mentioned earlier.[10–13]

Stage at Diagnosis and Survival

The clinical staging of any cancer defines the extent of disease in terms of anatomic spread, and is vital to the development of a treatment plan. It also provides the framework that permits comparison of treatment strategies, outcomes, and survival rates. The universally accepted TNM (Tumor, Node, Metastasis) staging system is used worldwide in staging malignant processes. Staging is site-specific and ranges from stage I (local disease) to stage IV (disseminated disease).

Of oral SCCs, 46% are diagnosed after the cancer has spread to locoregional lymph nodes (stage III); 35% have localized disease (stage I or II); 13% present with distantly disseminated metastatic disease (stage IV); and 6% present with unknown stage.[1] The corresponding 5-year survival rates are 55.1% (stage III), 77.2% (stage I and II), and 29.1% for disseminated disease (stage IV). This finding means that approximately 60% of oral SCCs are diagnosed at stage III or IV with a correspondingly low 5-year survival rate.

Statistics and detailed numbers notwithstanding, these data highlight 2 important facts:

A. Advances in treatment in the past several decades have not led to significant improvement in survival
B. Early diagnosis is a key factor in improving survival rate, thereby improving the morbidity and mortality associated with oral SCC.

Therefore, it is vital that dentists and hygienists, who serve as the gatekeepers of the oral cavity, understand the disease and recognize the clinical features of oral SCC and oral precancerous lesions.

CAUSE AND PATHOGENESIS

Oral SCC is a malignant neoplasm that arises from the squamous epithelium that lines the oral cavity. Familiarity with the general structure and function of squamous epithelium is essential for understanding the etiopathogenesis of oral SCC. The following review of the general pathogenetic mechanisms that drive malignant neoplastic progression provides the framework on which the various cause/risk factors of oral SCC are discussed.

Stratified squamous epithelium (unkeratinized/keratinized) lines the entire oral mucosal surface. Similar to any other type of epithelium, it rests on a complex fishnet-like basement membrane to which it is tethered by hemidesmosomes. Keratinocytes, the cells that serve as the functional units of all squamous epithelia, together form a meshwork of interconnected cells that comprise stratified squamous epithelium. The primary role of a keratinocyte is to proliferate and ascend from its origin in the basal-most stratum (basal cell layer) to the epithelial surface. As they ascend through the epithelial strata, keratinocytes are genetically programmed to differentiate, mature, undergo natural death, and finally leave a protective protein product, keratin, on the epithelial surface. Local homeostasis, especially in the basal and suprabasal epithelial layers, is tightly regulated by a series of genes that play critical roles in controlling the cell cycle of the keratinocyte (**Table 1**). Progression through the cell cycle is dependent on a combination of growth factors, growth suppressors, telomere length, and nutrition (vascular supply), and is regulated by checkpoint genes (eg, p53, p21, Rb), programmed cell death (apoptosis), local immune surveillance, and other factors. In addition, the components of the basement membrane (the structure that provides a natural barrier between the epithelium and the underlying superficial

Table 1
Pathogenetic mechanisms in oral carcinogenesis

Pathogenetic Mechanisms	GOF/LOF Mutations
A. Self-sufficiency in growth signals	A. Autocrine signaling (eg, GOF of EGF, TGFβ, KGF)
B. Insensitivity to antigrowth signals	B. LOF of tumor suppressors (eg, p16, p53, p21, CDK4/6)
C. Acquired capability to evade apoptosis	C. GOF of antiapoptotic genes or LOF of proapoptotic genes
D. Limitless replicative potential	D. Telomere lengthening (GOF of telomerase)
E. Sustained angiogenesis, stromal support	E. GOF mutations of angiogenic molecules (eg, VEGF, bFGF)
F. Tissue invasion and metastasis: Be independent of cell-cell interactions (loosen up) Acquire the ability to degrade the basement membrane and surrounding extracellular matrix Migration and locomotion Vascular/lymphatic dissemination and homing of tumor cells	F. Tissue invasion and metastasis: Mutations/ altered function of E-cadherins, β-catenin, keratins, actin cytoskeleton GOF produces proteolytic enzymes (eg, collagenases, MMPs, cathepsin D) and LOF of proteolytic inhibitors (eg, TIMPs) Abnormal proteolytic cleavage/folding of extracellular matrix proteins (eg, integrins, laminins, tenascin) Acquire the ability to survive in an unattached state Avoid local immune surveillance (decoy surface molecules) Migrate and home to vascular channels (chemokinesis) Survive mechanical shear (anoikis)

Abbreviations: anoikis, ability of cells to survive in dyshesive state; bFGF, basic fibroblast growth factor; EGF, epidermal growth factor; GOF, gain of function; LOF, loss of function; MMP, matrix met-alloprotease; TIMP, tissue inhibitor of matrix metalloprotease; TGF, transforming growth factor; VEGF, vascular endothelial growth factor.

submucosa [lamina propria] and serves as the foundation for the overlying epithelial strata) are maintained in a state of equilibrium by protease and antiprotease activity. Any lasting change (eg, acquired genetic defects, dysregulated immune function) that disturbs the local equilibrium potentially results in uncontrolled keratinocyte proliferation and/or loss of integrity of the epithelium-basement membrane relationship.

Normally, a range of inherent host regulatory/preventive mechanisms maintain orderly differentiation, growth, and integrity of the surface epithelium, so that to become a successful cancer cell an epithelial cell has to acquire certain properties that distinguish it from its surrounding normal counterparts. These distinguishing properties are acquired through mutations (see **Table 1**).[4,5,14]

A cell must acquire several mutations to be a successful cancer cell. Studies show that oral SCC, like most malignant tumors, results from a protracted sequence of events that recur repeatedly over many years. This finding is consistent with epidemiologic data that oral SCC is a disease that affects adults primarily. Several cancer progression models that focus on a few commonly affected molecules and genes have been proposed.[15,16] Nonetheless, the precise temporal sequence of mutations is different for each organ and tumor type, and varies from individual to individual.

RISK FACTORS

The genetic mutations leading to oral carcinogenesis may be spontaneous in some individuals. However, most are acquired, and are associated with predisposing or etiologic risk factors. Classic carcinogenesis experiments show the importance of risk factors and break them down into initiators and promoters that either inaugurate or advance permanent DNA damage. A single risk factor frequently can play both roles. Some of the risk factors/mutagens associated with oral SCC are discussed next.

Tobacco

Tobacco, the most common cause of human cancers, is responsible for ~85% of oral SCCs and ~90% of lung cancers.[17] Worldwide, cigarette smoking causes more than 5 million deaths annually. Numerous independent investigations in the past several decades have confirmed a link between oral SCC and tobacco smoking, including numerous case-control and cohort studies.[18-20] The proportion of smokers (~85%) among patients with oral SCC is nearly 3 times greater than the general population. In addition, studies show that the risk for a second primary carcinoma of the oral cavity/ aerodigestive tract is ~2 to 6 times greater in patients with a history of smoking. The number of potentially noxious/carcinogenic chemicals in tobacco smoke is extraordinary: it contains between 2000 and 4000 substances, 60 of which are identified carcinogens (nicotine, an alkaloid, is not a carcinogen but has been shown to be a potent addictive agent). Some substances generated by tobacco smoke that are recognized carcinogens include benzo[a]pyrene , TSNAs (tobacco-specific nitrosamines), phenol, and free radicals. Furthermore, studies consistently show a dose-response effect, with increased incidence of oral SCC related to the duration and frequency of smoking.[20-23] There is about a 20-fold risk of oral SCC in heavier tobacco smokers. Although increased smoking is related to increased risk for oral SCC, the risk for developing oral SCC does not necessarily diminish after cessation of smoking.[17,20,24]

As discussed earlier, the striking variations in oral SCC sites and incidence seen among different regional, cultural, and demographic groups are largely attributable to differences in the use and mode of delivery of tobacco. In the United States and much of the developed world cigarette smoking has been shown to have a linear dose-response carcinogenic effect. The risk for developing oral SCC remains the same, if not higher, in pipe and cigar smokers.[25] Smoking tobacco products like hookahs (water pipes), bidis (hand-rolled, filterless tobacco cigarettes), and chutta (reverse smoking) are associated with a similarly high risk for oral SCC.[26] Carcinogens from smoking that are released into the saliva tend to pool in the low-lying areas of the mouth and could account for the frequent occurrence of oral SCC along the lateral-ventral tongue and floor of the mouth.[9] In Southeast Asia and the Middle East, where habitual use of other carcinogenic substances is common, the oral cancer-prone sites are different from those cited earlier.[10] These patients' tumors tend to occur more often in the vestibular, gingival, and buccal mucosae, as a result of placement of noncombustible carcinogenic substances in direct and prolonged contact with these areas.

Smokeless tobacco use and its association with oral SCC has been the subject of several studies. Studies from Scandinavia have found that the use of Swedish snuff did not increase the risk of oral SCC.[27,28] However, some studies from the United States and around the world tell a different story. With the general upswing in snuff dipping and tobacco chewing, especially in the Southeastern United States, the incidence of oral SCC is higher than expected, especially in women.[29] A case-control study of 255 women in North Carolina showed a 50-fold increased risk for SCC of the gingiva and buccal mucosa in long-term snuff dippers.[30] The influence of smokeless tobacco on carcinogenesis seems to be associated with long-term use. Although studies often present conflicting opinions about smokeless tobacco, different risks are associated with different brands and products.[13,31] These differences are attributable to the presence/absence of additives, flavoring agents, and modifiers that enhance the carcinogenic potential of the smokeless tobacco. Most tobacco products consumed in Asia and Africa are unregulated and are often of the smokeless variety. Products such as paan (mixture of betel leaf, lime, tobacco, catechu, and areca nut), gutka (tobacco, areca nut), mishri (powdered tobacco that is rubbed on the gums), and chutta (clumps of tobacco that are either chewed or reverse smoked) are strong risk factors for oral SCC.

Tobacco smoking (past or present) remains the most consistent risk factor for oral SCC in the United States. Yet, with the increased use of smokeless tobacco, especially in women and young individuals and athletes, increased awareness of the potential risks of those products and association with oral SCC is a vital data point in screening for the disease. Any history of tobacco use (past or present; smoking/smokeless) must be viewed as a potential risk factor for oral SCC.

Alcohol

Alcohol is a well-recognized risk factor for several malignant neoplastic diseases, including oral SCC. It is recognized as a potent promoter of carcinogenesis. Ethanol is oxidized to acetaldehyde by alcohol dehydrogenase, releasing multiple free radicals. Although investigations that attempt to implicate alcohol alone as the main causative agent of oral SCC have yielded largely conflicting results, the correlation of alcohol with increased risk for oral SCC is indisputable.[17,32] The major clinical significance of alcohol consumption seems to be its ability to potentiate the carcinogenic effect of tobacco. The effect is at least additive and may be multiplicative in individuals with heavy alcohol consumption or at sites with the highest levels of alcohol exposure. Although the underlying mechanisms for this association are poorly understood, some proposed mechanisms include:

A. Dehydration effects of alcohol render the mucosa more susceptible to the carcinogens in tobacco

B. Alcohol activates carcinogens present in tobacco by a cytochrome p450-2E1–dependent toxin metabolism mechanism

C. Release of free radicals in the mucosa from local and hepatic alcohol metabolism results in mutagenesis.

Studies have shown that heavy alcohol consumption by itself or in addition to tobacco smoking produces about a 5-fold increased lifetime risk for developing oral SCC.[20,33,34] Studies looking into the risk associations between alcohol-containing mouth rinses and the development of oral cancer have not revealed any association. This finding was confirmed by an advisory panel convened by the US Food and Drug Administration (FDA) in 1996.

Therefore, although alcohol consumption by itself is not a proven oral SCC causative agent, it is recognized as a potent contributory/independent risk factor when consumed in large quantities and in combination with tobacco smoking.

Human Papilloma Virus

Human papilloma viruses (HPVs) are epitheliotropic DNA viruses with more than 130 identified genotypes. Several strains of HPV (HPV 4,6,11,13,31) are known to cause common viral warts (squamous papilloma, verruca vulgaris) of the skin and mucosal surfaces in children, youths, and adults. The strains HPV 16 and 18 have been closely associated with and implicated in cervical cancers; they are often referred to as the high-risk strains of HPV (HR HPVs). The oncogenic potential of HR HPVs has been attributed to their ability to insert their early genes (E6, E7) into the genome of the host cell, thereby abrogating the critical function of tumor-suppressor and cell-cycle regulatory genes pRb and p53. This situation leads to deregulation of the cell cycle, and impaired apoptotic mechanisms and DNA repair, all of which contribute to malignant progression.[35]

Several recent investigations have reported on the association of HR HPVs and a subset of oropharyngeal SCCs.[36,37] These studies uncovered a wide range of viral prevalence (0%–100%) in the tumors reviewed. This finding may in large part be attributable to the natural presence of both HR HPVs and other HPV strains in normal mucosa.[38] Nonetheless, in the literature much confusion concerning the role of HPV in oral carcinogenesis has been generated by pooling SCCs from the oral cavity proper and the pharynx and larynx into a single large grouping of head and neck cancer. This tendency to pool disparate site statistics into a single category of disease has led to misunderstanding about the role of HPV relative to carcinogenesis of the oral cavity, because it seems that there are recognized sites in the oropharynx that are more susceptible than the oral cavity mucosa to the oncogenic influence of HPVs. Specific areas in the pharynx and larynx, including the tonsils (ie, squamous-columnar junctions of the crypts and glottides), are believed to harbor greatest susceptibility to HPV because of ready exposure of their basal epithelial cells. (These microenvironments are anatomically similar to the HPV-susceptible transformation zone in the cervix.)

HR HPVs are associated with a subset of SCCs of the pharynx, larynx, and tonsillar tissues in patients who are nonsmokers and nondrinkers.[36,37] The subset of HR HPVs-associated oropharyngeal SCCs have been shown to be more responsive to radiochemotherapy, and have more favorable treatment outcomes compared with tobacco/alcohol associated SCCs. However, a similar association has not been established between HPV16/18 and oral cavity SCC. Although the presence of E6/E7 HPV transcripts can be noted in some oral SCCs, these early proteins have also been found in perfectly normal oral mucosal epithelial cells.[38] That finding raises the question as to whether HR HPV transcripts present in oral epithelial cells indicate HPV as an agent of carcinogenesis or as an innocent bystander. The tendency to group some HPV-positive oropharyngeal cancers with oral cavity cancers likely accounts for the purported but apparently mistaken notion that oral cancers in general are associated with HPV.

HPV is a common virus associated with many benign oral lesions (verruca vulgaris, squamous papilloma, Heck disease). HPV infection is associated with some oropharyngeal SCCs, but HR HPVs (HPV 16/18) do not seem to play an identified role in oral SCC, and the alleged connection has not been confirmed. Tobacco and alcohol remain the most well-established oral SCC risk factors.

Genetic Susceptibility

The relationship between oral SCC and exposure to tobacco and alcohol is well recognized. It is also well known that only a fraction of smokers and drinkers develop oral SCC. The incidence of oral cancer in individuals less than age 40 years who have no known risk factors has been increasing in recent years and may be attributable to underlying genetic susceptibility.[39–41] As discussed earlier, individuals with underlying defects of key molecules/genes responsible for maintaining local homeostasis are predisposed to developing oral SCC when exposed to initiating/promoting agents like tobacco and alcohol. Emerging studies show inherent differences between individuals[38] in their DNA repair mechanisms, cell cycle control/apoptosis mechanisms, and/or immune surveillance mechanisms, among others. If future population-based studies successfully identify underlying genetic defects that predispose individuals to developing oral SCC, the information gleaned could substantially improve primary/secondary prevention and early detection.

Radiation

Exposure to ionizing radiation is a well-recognized risk factor for nonmelanoma skin cancers (basal cell carcinomas and SCCs). Ultraviolet (UV) radiation is known to cause DNA damage and mutations in critical DNA repair mechanisms (p53, MDM2) and is a known risk factor for actinic cheilitis and SCC of the lip. However, there is no association between exposure to ionizing radiation and the development of intraoral SCC. Therefore, as discussed earlier, it is important to exclude SCCs of the lip in our discussion of intraoral SCCs. Therapeutic irradiation of the head and neck does not seem to induce second primary SCCs. In years past it was believed that therapeutic irradiation of oral verrucous carcinomas was associated with a high transformation rate to conventional and anaplastic oral SCC. However, more recent analysis reveals this claim not to be true. Therapeutic irradiation of verrucous carcinoma has been shown to yield results comparable with those obtained with conventional SCC.[42–44]

CLINICAL CONSIDERATIONS: ORAL CANCERS AND PRECANCEROUS LESIONS

Familiarity with the profile of a patient who has oral cancer, including the risk factors as described earlier, and the composite classic clinical features of an oral cancer and its precursor lesions, enhances the clinician's ability to diagnose and intercept evolving carcinomas.

SCC: Clinical Features

Clinical presentation
Who is the classic patient with oral cancer? Because the process of malignant transformation is notoriously protracted, oral SCC is a disease of individuals 45 years of age or older; it is less common in younger persons (see **Fig. 1**). There is usually a past or

active history of tobacco use. Risk for developing a second upper aerodigestive tract malignancy in patients who have oral cancer who continue to smoke is also significantly magnified. The implications of smoking go even further: long considered a male-dominated disease, in recent decades the male/female ratio for oral cancer has been narrowing toward parity. This situation is likely attributable in part to the more socially acceptable use of tobacco among women that began during the period just before World War II and persisted, thus effecting the shifting gender predilection for oral cancer. Tobacco exposure combined with alcohol ingestion seems to heighten the risk for disease. Although moderate intake of alcohol alone was believed to function not as a direct carcinogen but instead as a promoter or potentiating agent for cancer development, recent epidemiologic investigation suggests that chronic ingestion of alcohol at high levels can be an independent risk factor for oral cancer.[20,32] In unusual cases of oral SCC in individuals less than 40 years of age, epidemiologic studies have not disclosed a significant association between chronic alcohol or tobacco use. Individuals with a prior history of oral cancer or a documented history of one or more precancerous oral lesions are at significant risk for recurrent disease or second primary carcinomas in the oral cavity and upper aerodigestive tract.[45]

Location

Where are oral cancers found? Most SCCs do not occur randomly within the oral cavity. Knowing their most likely locations is vital, not only for case finding (ie, establishing a diagnosis when abnormal signs and symptoms are obvious) but also with regard to screening for oral cancer (ie, pointedly examining for suspicious findings in otherwise asymptomatic individuals or population groups at risk for the disease). Earlier US studies of large numbers of small, localized primary oral SCCs revealed that most of the tumors appeared to favor certain intraoral locations more than others.[8,9] These so-called oral cancer-prone sites include the lateral and ventral aspects of the tongue, the floor of mouth, and the soft palate-uvula-tonsillar pillar complexes. All of the latter locations are surfaced by unkeratinized mucosa. Presumably, in these particular areas carcinogens dissolved in saliva encounter a thin mucosal barrier that permits their prolonged contact with and ready access to the surface epithelial squamous cells.

Appearance

Classic (conventional) oral SCC in most cases presents itself on one of the aforementioned cancer-predilection sites as an ulcerated white, or red, or red and white mass, usually with nonhomogeneous (eg, corrugated, verrucous, pebbly, or nodular) surface topography (**Fig. 2**A–E). There may or may not be pain or paresthesia. On palpation the mass feels indurated; its extent may be difficult to define because of both the endophytic and circumferential growth patterns of the invasive process. Depending on the location, tumor invasion can and frequently does eventuate in loss of mobility or tethering fixation of neighboring anatomic structures in the path of the tumor. This situation can result in functional compromise relative to speech, mastication, and deglutition. Invasion into adjacent or underlying maxillary or mandibular bone can result in unconfined lytic destruction of the alveolar bone and periodontium attended by dramatic tooth mobility. Tumor infiltration of the inferior alveolar nerve is associated with pain and paresthesia (**Fig. 3**).

Verrucous Carcinoma: A Low-Grade Variant of Oral SCC

Verrucous carcinoma is a low-grade type of well-differentiated SCC with distinctive clinicopathologic features. Although there had been speculation about an etiologic

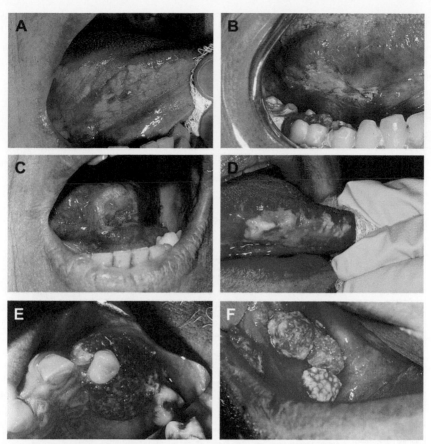

Fig. 2. Clinical features of oral SCC and verrucous carcinoma. (*A*) SCC, right ventral-lateral tongue. Surrounding tongue surface shows extensive, contiguous erythroleukoplakic change that extended into floor of mouth, lingual aspect of mandibular right alveolar mucosa, and gingiva. (*B*) SCC, right posterior ventral-lateral tongue. Patient had been aware of a painless ulcer in the area for nearly 1 year. The patient's dentist did not notice the lesion but had recently placed an amalgam restoration in the lower right second molar tooth. (*C*) SCC, ventral anterior tongue, causing limitation of tongue mobility. Note tethering of tongue to floor of mouth. (*D*) Erythroleukoplakia, recurrent, right lateral tongue. The patient had already had 3 similar-appearing lesions excised previously in this location. Histopathologic examination of the excisional biopsies showed varying degrees of intraepithelial dysplasia with occasional foci of superficially invasive SCC. (*E*) SCC, papillary features, maxillary gingiva. Note leukoplakic changes on gingiva anterior to mass. (*F*) Verrucous carcinoma, right buccal mucosa.

role for HPV in the development of verrucous carcinoma, there is no consistent evidence to support this conjecture.[46] Exposure to smoked tobacco products, particularly pipes and cigar smoking, seems to be contributory in some patients. Another contributing factor is advancing age, because verrucous carcinoma does seem to favor older individuals, including elderly women with negligible smoking histories. The behavior of the tumor is more indolent than that of conventional SCC, in that it spreads superficially and slowly and rarely if ever metastasizes. The growth pattern of verrucous carcinoma tends to be more exophytic than infiltrative: unlike

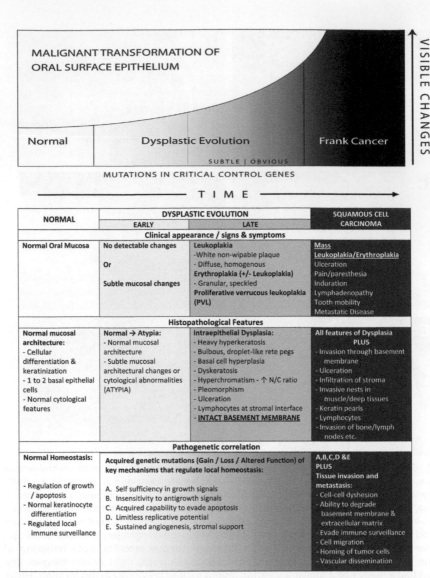

Fig. 3. Clinical, histologic, and pathogenetic molecular progression from normal oral mucosa to SCC. Malignant transformation of oral surface epithelium is a result of accumulation of mutations in critical control genes occurs over a period of time (years to decades). Note that the underlying genetic defects do not show obvious clinical and histopathologic phenotypic changes until later in the process. (1) Clinical features observed during the progression from normal oral mucosal to dysplasia to oral SCC. (2) Characteristic histopathologic features observed during oral cancer progression from normal to atypical to dysplasia and oral SCC. (3) Acquired genetic defects seen in cancerous cells during the progression from normal to dysplastic to oral SCC (refer to **Table 1** for details). (*Data from* Eisenberg E. Frozen section examination of the margins for resection of squamous cell carcinoma of the lower lip. J Oral Maxillofacial Surg 2003;61:896.)

conventional SCC, the pathognomonically broad, bulbous rete pegs of the advancing tumor seem to push down into the underlying stroma rather than invade it in an unfettered, insidious manner. Clinically, verrucous carcinoma spreads circumferentially along the mucosal surface from its respective epicenter, favoring locations that include the buccal, vestibular, and gingival-alveolar mucosae in either arch as points of origin. (These sites are also the ones conventional SCCs seem to favor in individuals who inveterately apply noncombustible carcinogenic substances [eg, betel, gutka, smokeless tobacco] to the oral mucosa.) Verrucous carcinomas show a strikingly exophytic white, or red and white, shaggy carpetlike warty configuration (see **Fig. 2**F). With time, a verrucous carcinoma can undergo transformation to a more clinicopathologically conventional SCC, with more locally destructive, infiltrative growth and potential for metastasis.[46]

Oral Premalignant Lesions: Clinical Features

The spectrum of clinical features described earlier comprises a kind of snapshot taken late in the life history of an individual oral cancer (see **Fig. 3**). However, before the emergence of a frank squamous cell (or a verrucous) carcinoma, clinically visible preinvasive (precancerous) oral mucosal surface changes are frequently observed at sites of future tumor presentation. This finding suggests that clinically manifest precancerous lesions augur a risk for cancer development. The recognized precancerous mucosal alterations present as clinical findings typically described as leukoplakia, erythroplakia (a red, velvety-textured mucosal patch) or, when combined, speckled (or erythro-) leukoplakia (see **Figs. 2** and **3**). Frequently these changes associated with preinvasion are also seen on mucosal surfaces adjacent to and contiguous with a carcinoma, and may be seen to extend for some distance beyond the region immediately proximal to a tumor. The widespread nature of the mucosal changes as described here embodies clinical evidence of the field effect[47] from mutations that affect the entire region. However, whether or not an individual leukoplakic or erythroplakic lesion is a precancerous lesion (which implies that it harbors potential for progression to carcinoma) is indicated by its histopathologic features.

LEUKOPLAKIA AND ERYTHROPLAKIA

What is leukoplakia? In our observation, leukoplakia is a term that is liberally applied by many to indicate any white oral mucosal lesion. Some have also used the term leukoplakia generically as a specific diagnosis referable to oral cancer or precancer. This situation has generated considerable diagnostic confusion and misunderstanding. Although some leukoplakias (and erythroplakias) are clinical precursor lesions of oral SCC, not all leukoplakic (or erythroplakic) lesions are premalignant. Hence, it is not appropriate to use the terms leukoplakia and erythroplakia as synonyms for precancer. It is also inappropriate to apply the term leukoplakia to any and all white lesions. Therefore, it is incumbent on clinicians to be able to distinguish leukoplakic from nonleukoplakic white lesions, and to recognize the profile of suspicious white (and/or red) lesions in contrast to those that are innocent.

The World Health Organization (WHO) defines leukoplakia as "...a predominantly white patch that cannot be characterized clinically or histopathologically as any other definable lesion."[48] (Erythroplakia is defined in a manner similar to the manner in which leukoplakia is defined.) In our view, this characterization is diagnostically confusing and ripe for misapplication. In the strictly clinical sense, all leukoplakic lesions are white, but not all white lesions are leukoplakias. Leukoplakia correctly defined is "a white non-wipable mucosal patch or plaque that cannot be attributed clinically to any other diagnosable condition."[49–51] So what is leukoplakia?

1. "A white non-wipable mucosal plaque…": the term leukoplakia refers to and should be reserved solely for a white nonwipable mucosal plaque, which means that it is epithelial and keratotic in nature, rather than representative of pseudomembranous candidal elements, necrotic matter, or myriad other surface debris.

2. "…..that cannot be attributed clinically to any other diagnosable condition.": For example, a white nonwipable plaque on an intraoral location that is naturally trauma-protected rather than subject to irritation, and whose history is negative for trauma or irritation is not readily suggestive clinically of a benign reactive hyper-keratosis. It is thus diagnostically indeterminate on strictly clinical grounds and can be designated as leukoplakia. On the other hand, a white lesion is not considered leukoplakia if it is clinically recognizable as a particular condition or disease entity, such as linea alba, leukoedema, lichen planus, or a mucocutaneous manifestation of lupus erythematosus; or if by history and clinical distribution it is obviously a manifestation of a specific genetic condition such as the genokeratosis, white sponge nevus.

In particular, white nonwipable lesions on cancer-prone sites where there is no obvious or identifiable source of friction are classic examples of leukoplakia (**Fig. 4**A–D). In patients with a known history of exposure to carcinogen, a clinically

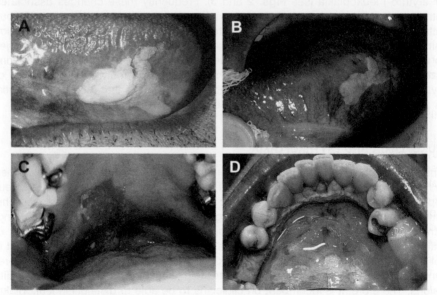

Fig. 4. Clinical features of oral precancerous lesions (epithelial dysplasias). (*A*) Leukoplakia, left lateral tongue. Note the variation in thickness of the lesion and its extent posteriorly and inferiorly. (*B*) Pebbly-appearing leukoplakia, left lateral tongue. This example of field cancerization developed in the same patient whose carcinomatous and dysplastic lesions on contralateral tongue surface are shown in **Fig. 2**. The patient eventually developed another SCC on the right lingual gingival, with invasion into the mandible. (*C*) Extensive erythroleukoplakia, right soft palate. Histopathology revealed carcinoma in situ and foci of mild to moderate dysplasia. (*D*) PVL. Initial presentation was on the lower anterior lingual gingival.

indeterminate white lesion irrespective of location may be regarded as leukoplakia. Thus, the designation leukoplakia is reserved for use as an exclusively provisional clinical designation rather than a definitive diagnosis.

Representative tissue sampling (incisional or excisional biopsy) followed by histopathologic evaluation is necessary to determine the specific diagnosis. Once a representative tissue biopsy has been obtained, reviewed at the microscope, and a diagnosis rendered based on the constellation of histopathologic findings observed, the designation leukoplakia is then replaced by the definitive diagnosis revealed from that analysis. Histopathologic diagnoses range from benign hyperkeratotic lesions in most cases, to premalignant lesions (epithelial dysplasia/carcinoma in situ) and carcinomas, in fewer instances. Erythroplakic mucosal lesions are even more likely than leukoplakias to show premalignant changes on microscopic examination. A histopathologic diagnosis of leukoplakia (or erythroplakia) is incomprehensible. Therefore, given the diagnostic specificity gleaned from microscopic evaluation, it is difficult to understand the WHO's rationale for including "histopathology" in its current definition of either leukoplakia or erythroplakia.

Proliferative Verrucous Leukoplakia

Proliferative verrucous leukoplakia (PVL) is a progressive, widespread and often multifocal form of leukoplakia or erythroleukoplakia.[51] PVL lesions spread circumferentially and often relentlessly over the course of many years. They have a tendency to transform to either SCC or verrucous carcinoma and, given sufficient time, many PVLs develop into malignancies that likely recur.[52–55] Mortality for PVL-associated cancer reportedly is 39% to 43%. Distinct from other forms of oral leukoplakia and SCC, a causal linkage between PVL lesions and tobacco or alcohol is not consistent. Although there had been speculation about a possible etiologic role for HPV in the propagation and progression of PVL, there is no consistent evidence to support that contention,[56,57] so the underlying cause for PVL remains unknown.

HISTOPATHOLOGY OF ORAL SCC AND PREMALIGNANT LESIONS

The gold-standard technique for definitive diagnosis of oral SCC and premalignant (dysplastic) epithelial lesions involves microscopic examination of a representative tissue sample obtained through an incisional (or excisional) biopsy. Tissue biopsy rather than cytologic sampling permits a thorough evaluation of the epithelial cytomorphology of the lesion, its architecture, and its relationship to underlying structures. In some instances, a tissue biopsy also permits an evaluation of the surface epithelium adjacent to the clinically abnormal-appearing tissue. Observance of epithelial architecture (topography) is a key element of microscopic interpretation, especially when the concern is oral cancer or precancer. Correlation of both cell-to-cell and topographic relations is critical for proper assessment and is unquestionably superior to any other alternative diagnostic technologies. Histopathologic interpretation of a tissue biopsy yields a specific diagnosis.

Epithelial Dysplasia

Epithelial dysplasia refers to a composite of cytomorphologic and architectural changes in squamous epithelium that are recognized as indicative of premalignant status, that is, invasive potential.[58] By definition dysplasia is an exclusively intraepithelial lesion (ie, it is confined to the region above the basement membrane). A spectrum of findings constitutes dysplastic change; every dysplastic lesion exhibits at least 2 or more features reflective of maturational abnormality among those enumerated here (see **Fig. 3**).

On low-power examination, the overall topography of dysplastic surface epithelium deviates from normal. Rete pegs are blunt, often broad and bulbous, round, or tear-drop-shaped. The basal cells may line up in a regimental, picket-fencelike arrangement, with strikingly hyperchromatic, elongated nuclei. There is stratification disarray, with an increase in number of basaloid-appearing cells that may extend superiorly into the stratum spinosum region. Nuclear pleomorphism, hyperchromatism, dyskeratosis (eg, premature and individual cell keratinization, keratin pearl formation), apoptosis, and increased numbers of mitotic figures, normal or abnormal, beyond the strictly basal cell stratum are among the possible cytomorphologic irregularities observed in epithelial dysplasia. There may be evident loss of cell-to-cell cohesion (**Fig. 5A–D**).

Pathologists often characterize individual dysplastic lesions as mild (subtle), moderate, or severe (carcinoma in situ) in histopathologic degree depending on the extent of architectural, cellular, and maturational abnormality observed from the basal cell layer inferiorly, to the epithelial surface superiorly. Some regard mild dysplasia as a falsely positive epithelial lesion that is less likely than severe dysplasia or carcinoma in situ to progress to frank malignancy. However, that is not the way disease happens in practice: given time, even a mildly dysplastic lesion can and certainly has succeeded in evolving to invasive cancer. However, neither the likelihood that any single dysplastic lesion advances to a frankly invasive SCC nor the rate of such transformation can be predicted with certainty based on the degree of dysplastic change observed at the microscope. Therefore, irrespective of degree, a diagnosis of dysplasia should alert the clinician that there is a recognized risk for such progression, and that ongoing clinical vigilance is mandatory.

Epithelial Atypia

More modest deviations from normal epithelial architecture or cytomorphology revealed on light microscopic examination of tissue are designated as atypical features (epithelial atypia).[58] A diagnosis of epithelial atypia frequently presents a diagnostic challenge to both the pathologist and the clinician, because it could represent either an unusual, albeit fundamentally benign tissue response to an inflammatory, infectious, or some other unspecified stimulus; or it may indicate evolving dysplastic change. In many cases it might not be possible to distinguish the benign epithelial atypias from those that represent a stage in the process of dysplastic progression. There are no known molecular/genetic markers that can demarcate benign from dysplastic epithelial atypias. Nonetheless, history, clinical information, and composite histopathologic findings combined are the essential elements necessary to guide the clinician's approach to an individual patient's atypical epithelial lesion. Epithelial lesions diagnostically designated as atypical must be followed regularly, and be rebiopsied propitiously if or when clinical and/or historical circumstances indicate such need. Clinical evidence of extension and/or heterogeneity in surface character (thickening, corrugation, pebbly texture, color, erosion, ulceration, nodularity) of the preexisting lesion are indications for rebiopsy.

SCC

What are the histopathologic features of SCC? An individual SCC may be classified as well-, moderately-, or poorly differentiated, depending on the degree of keratinization and recognizable squamous epithelial characteristics it shows. Malignant epithelium shows stratification disarray. There is surface hyperkeratosis or acanthosis alternating

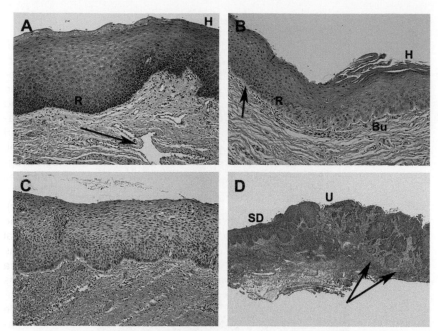

Fig. 5. Histopathologic features of oral precancerous lesions (oral intraepithelial dysplasia) and progression to SCC. (*A*) Mild epithelial dysplasia. The oral epithelium shows surface hyperkeratosis (H, white clinical appearance) and mild architectural disarray in the lower third of the epithelium: basal cell hyperchromasia, regimentation (R) and hyperplasia, nuclear enlargement and broad, blunt rete pegs. Note the dilated blood vessels (*arrow*) in the submucosa (clinically red and white). (*B*) Mild to moderate dysplasia. Dysplastic changes extend to the midpoint of the epithelium and are characterized by surface hyperkeratosis (H), blunting and budding of rete pegs (Bu), basal cell hyperchromasia, enlargement and regimentation (R). Note that the epithelium on the left (*arrow*) is not as hyperkeratinized (not clinically obvious) but likely harbors the same genetic mutations that led to the architectural disarray seen on the right side. (*C*) Moderate to severe dysplasia. Dysplastic changes extend from the midpoint and above to involve full thickness of epithelium characterized by broad, blunt rete pegs, basal cell hyperplasia (>two-thirds thickness), nuclear enlargement, lack of normal differentiation, and a mild chronic inflammatory infiltrate in the submucosa. (*D*) Infiltrative SCC. Low-power scanning showing progression from severe dysplasia (SD) to infiltrative SCC. Observe the central area of ulceration (U), infiltrative nests of tumor in the underlying submucosa (*arrows*) and accompanying inflammatory infiltrate.

with epithelial atrophy, and ulceration is frequently observed. Attendant cytologic abnormalities can vary from tumor to tumor, but they include at least several of the following: nuclear enlargement, hyperchromatism, cellular and nuclear pleomorphism, dyskeratosis (ie, individual cell keratinization, keratin pearl formation), acantholysis, apoptosis, and increased mitotic activity, often with abnormal mitoses involving basal and suprabasal strata. The rete pegs are highly irregular in shape, depth, and number. Irrespective of the number of cytomorphologic abnormalities observed, the histopathologic hallmark of malignancy is evidence that the basement membrane (ie, the epithelial-stromal boundary) has been breached, permitting invasion of transformed dysplastic (preinvasive) surface epithelium into the underlying submucosa (see **Fig. 5**D; **Fig. 6**). With violation of that anatomic boundary, the infiltrating tumor has access to vasculature and lymphatic channels. This situation creates potential for

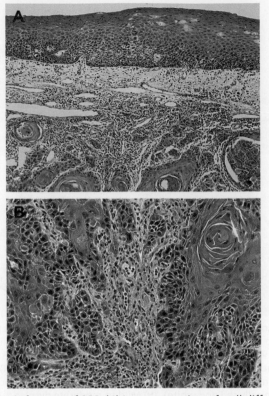

Fig. 6. Histopathologic features of SCC. (*A*) Low-power view of well-differentiated SCC. The submucosa contains numerous infiltrative nests of neoplastic epithelium with keratin pearl formation and central necrosis, inflammatory infiltrates, and vascular ectasia. Note that the overlying epithelium that represents a portion of the tumor margin exhibits mild epithelial dysplasia. (*B*) High-power view of well-differentiated SCC. Neoplastic nests show keratin pearl formation, dyskeratosis, cellular pleomorphism, and mitotic figures, and surrounding tissue is chronically inflamed.

tumor metastasis via lymphangitic spread. Necrosis, chronic inflammation, vascular ectasia, and hemorrhage are also frequently observed. Neurotropism (ie, the demonstrated proclivity of the malignant neoplastic elements for invasion of nerves and perineural spaces) is a particularly ominous prognostic indicator for oral SCC.

ADJUNCTIVE SCREENING AND DIAGNOSTIC TOOLS

Poor survival rates in patients with oral SCC are largely the result of advanced disease at the time of diagnosis, with more than 60% of patients presenting in stages III and IV. It is disturbing that these statistics have remained unchanged for several decades given the accessibility of the oral cavity to direct visual and tactile examination. The failure or inability of clinicians to recognize clinically suspicious lesions as early as possible is one of the factors responsible for the dismal statistics. Therefore it is imperative to raise public awareness and also provide health professionals with the education and training to recognize clinically suspicious oral lesions. However, it is also important to acknowledge that oral cancer is a genetic disease in which epithelial tissue acquires an abnormal genotype long before it is manifested as a clinically obvious abnormality. Thus, the biology of oral cancer development itself likely contributes to clinicians' failure to consistently identify suspicious lesions as early as possible (see **Fig. 3**). In response to the need for improvement in early detection, several diagnostic aids intended to help in the identification and assessment of oral lesions have been developed and made available to clinicians in recent years. We discuss and evaluate the efficacy of these screening and diagnostic aids, and compare them to standard oral examination.

Standard Oral Examination

Standard oral examination of visually accessible areas of the oral cavity under incandescent light has long been the mainstay of screening for oral cancer. For decades, studies have shown that thorough visual and palpatory oral examination supplemented by evaluation of the patient's history of exposure to risk factors are effective for detecting suspicious oral lesions.

Nonetheless, conventional oral examination does have some limitations. Although the classic clinical presentation of an oral premalignant lesion (a leukoplakic or erythroleukoplakic patch or persistent ulcer that cannot be diagnosed as any other clinical condition) is well known, only a modest proportion of leukoplakic lesions show precancerous changes or SCC on microscopic examination. Of those lesions found to have histologically premalignant features, not all progress to oral SCC. Thus, neither clinical examination nor histopathologic diagnosis can reliably predict which biopsy-proven dysplastic lesion is likely to progress to oral SCC. Another limitation of conventional oral examination relates to the biology of oral cancer evolution and the field effect[47,59]: oral cavity epithelium that is already transformed genotypically but that does not yet exhibit phenotypic (clinical) evidence of surface mucosal abnormality appears clinically normal (see **Fig. 3**). Therefore, conventional examination may not be capable of readily identifying all potentially premalignant lesions. Several of the new technologies attempt to address these inadequacies.

Brush Cytology

The brush biopsy (Oral CDx, OralCDx Laboratories, Inc, Suffern, NY, USA) is a technique for cytologic sampling that has been available since 1999. It is intended for use as a case-finding tool for investigating clinical oral lesions that would normally not be subjected to conventional (incisional) biopsy because their clinical presentation carries a low profile of suspicion for SCC.[60] Oral cytology specimens retrieved through brush-biopsy sampling are examined and interpreted by using both a computer algorithm and a human cytopathologist's analysis combined. Three possible results are reported from the analysis: negative (for cytologic abnormality); atypical (denotes deviations from normal cytology that arouse concern about, but are not unequivocal evidence of precancer [epithelial dysplasia] or cancer); and positive (findings suggestive of dysplasia or carcinoma). Although atypical and positive are abnormal results they are not definitive diagnoses. The latter 2 results therefore require further investigation, which in most cases is clinical reevaluation and a tissue biopsy, the gold-standard technique for definitive diagnosis of oral mucosal lesions. It is not appropriate to repeat the cytobrush sampling rather than perform a tissue biopsy as follow-up to an abnormal cytobrush result.

Unlike the results of conventional tissue biopsy analysis, brush cytology does not yield specific diagnoses. Even when the brush cytology result is negative it is impossible to establish a specific diagnosis solely through analysis of disarticulated cells, without the ability to evaluate epithelial architecture, epithelial-connective tissue relationships, and cell-to-cell relationships. In our experience, many tissue biopsies performed following atypical cytobrush results have shown epithelial atypia in association with intense inflammatory infiltration within the underlying submucosa. Such atypia can be interpreted as an unusual reactive and fundamentally benign epithelial response, driven by inflammatory stimulation rather than demonstrative of dysplastic evolution.

From published reports, the overall efficacy of oral brush cytology is questionable for reasons that are carefully summarized by Lingen and colleagues[61] in their critical evaluation of diagnostic detection aids for oral cancerous lesions. Some of the studies these investigators reviewed involved large numbers of subjects and included clinically innocent as well as clinically suspicious lesions. In several of the studies that examined the sensitivity and specificity of brush cytology for evaluation of precancerous oral lesions, only clinically suspicious lesions were both brush sampled and subjected to scalpel biopsy. However, brush cytology was not intended for clinically suspicious lesions. Because the technique is aimed at those lesions considered clinically innocent, it is critical to be able to correlate cytologic findings with tissue biopsy findings from such lesions. In another large study of clinically innocuous lesions subjected to brush sampling, tissue biopsies were not performed on all of the subjects, nor were they obtained in all cases in which the cytobrush results were abnormal. Lingen's group as well as other reviewers of the various studies[62–65] emphasize that until an adequate cohort of subjects with innocuous lesions that have been sampled both by brush for cytology and by scalpel for tissue biopsy is studied and reported, the technique may be regarded as promising, but no absolute conclusions about its efficacy can be drawn.

The cytobrush technique has served to raise clinicians' awareness of the need to scrupulously examine the entire mucosal surface of the oral cavity and to follow up on suspicious findings. This technique holds promise for future applications, perhaps in combination with as yet unidentified biomarkers definitively linked to dysplasia and carcinoma.

Toluidine Blue

Toluidine blue (tolonium chloride) has been used for decades for detection of mucosal abnormalities in the oral cavity and other mucosal sites. It is a metachromatic dye that purportedly binds to tissues that are actively proliferating, by staining nucleic acids within the dividing cells. Active tissue proliferation is not limited to malignancy exclusively; it is also encountered in inflammatory and reactive processes. Although not FDA approved for oral cancer screening in the United States, toluidine blue has been used in other parts of the world as a screening tool for oral cancer. It has also been used by some surgeons as a guide for selecting sites for obtaining representative biopsy specimens from extensive clinically suspicious oral mucosal lesions. Some surgeons have also found it useful for demarcating the extent of a biopsy-proven dysplastic lesion as they attempt to determine surgical excision borders.

Several studies have looked into the efficacy of toluidine blue as a screening tool for precancer and cancer. A consistent finding across multiple studies is the ability of toluidine blue to disclose oral SCC with high sensitivity, ranging from 92% to 100%.[61] However, with regard to the ability of toluidine blue to disclose dysplastic lesions in previously undiagnosed patients there have been mixed results. Fewer than 50% of dysplastic lesions stained positive with toluidine blue, which precludes any real benefit for early SCC detection. Further compromising its efficacy as a screening tool is the tendency of the dye to stain common benign conditions such as nonspecific ulcerations, epithelial hyperplasias, chronic frictional keratoses, and other similar lesions, thus resulting in a high proportion of false-positive results. Gray and colleagues[66] concluded that toluidine blue was not an effective screening tool to be used in a primary care setting, such as a general dentist's office. However, the value of tolu-idine blue is probably greatest as a treatment planning adjunct once a diagnosis of dysplasia or carcinoma has been established through a conventional biopsy.

Tissue-reflectance Systems (ViziLite and Microlux)

Tissue-reflectance detection systems for oral examination, ViziLite (Zila Pharmaceuti-cals Inc, Phoenix, AZ, USA) and Microlux (AdDent Inc, Danbury, CT, USA), were devel-oped from chemiluminescent systems similar to the ones that have been used for the detection of cervical neoplasia. The design and rationale for use of these systems is based on the principle that on exposure to acetic acid, clusters of rapidly proliferating cells (ie, cells with activated nucleic acid), preferentially reflect the low-energy blue-white light emitted by the hand-held light sources of the systems. To use these systems, patients rinse first with a 1% acetic acid solution. This procedure is followed by direct examination of the oral mucous membranes under the blue-white light source. ViziLite uses a disposable light system, whereas Microlux is a multiuse system that uses a blue-white light generated by fiber optics or light-emitting diodes. Under such illumination, normal mucosal surfaces appear light blue, whereas abnormal proliferative areas of the epithelium are acetowhite. Presumably this effect discloses areas suspicious for precancer or cancer.

Several studies that explore the efficacy of tissue-reflectance systems for the detec-tion of precancerous lesions have been conducted.[61] A consistent finding across some studies using ViziLite was the ability of the system to disclose a variety of diverse oral lesions. Among the lesions detected and confirmed with tissue biopsies were common benign entities such as leukoedema, lichen planus, linea alba, benign hyper-keratosis, and fibrous hyperplasia.[67] However, all of these lesions were readily visible without the aid of ViziLite. Although the reported sensitivity of ViziLite was consistently high across studies ($\sim$95%–100%), its diagnostic specificity was consistently low (0%–10%). With consistently low positive predictive values across studies, it seems that ViziLite and similar tissue-reflectance systems do not provide any added advan-tage over standard visual examination. There is little evidence in the published studies to support the use of either ViziLite or Microlux tissue-reflectance systems in the detection of oral precancer and cancer.[61]

The ViziLite system has recently been combined with the toluidine blue system and is now available as ViziLite Plus. In 2 published studies looking at the efficacy of Vizi-Lite Plus, the combined system is reported to improve the detection rate of precan-cerous lesions, with increased specificity and positive predictive values. However, the studies were conducted on lesions already identified on standard (ie, unaided) visual examination. Although ViziLite Plus enhanced $\sim$60% of visually identified lesions, it did not reveal any additional lesions. Thus, although the value of ViziLite Plus as a screening/diagnostic tool is questionable, a potential application could be its use as a treatment planning adjunct for managing lesions that have been proved to be premalignant or malignant.

VELscope: A Tissue Autofluorescence System

The VELscope (LED Dental Inc, British Columbia, Canada) is a hand-held device used to assist direct visualization of tissues. It relies on the well-known phenomenon of tissue autofluorescence (TA). TA is produced by naturally occurring fluorophores within all cells that yield reflective and absorptive patterns that are unique to each tissue. As an example, when viewed through a selective narrow-band filter, normal oral mucosal surface epithelium emits pale green autofluorescence. Based on the principle described earlier, the VELscope generates a 400- to 460-nm blue excitation light, which is shined directly on the oral mucosa. Any tissue abnormality or barrier that prevents or reduces rebound from the blue excitation light results in decreased fluorescence. Therefore, areas with abnormal proliferation (as seen in premalignancy and malignancy) appear darker compared with surrounding healthy tissue.

Although in theory the device seems to have the potential to detect epithelial dysplasia in otherwise normal-appearing oral mucosal tissue, no randomized, controlled studies have investigated its efficacy as a primary screening tool.[61] Most of the studies have been performed in patients who already had a history of oral epithelial dysplasia or SCC identified by standard visual examination. The few reports that showed the ability of VELscope to identify dysplastic lesions that were not seen on standard visual examination were reports of anecdotal observations alone, rather than controlled, randomized trials.

A potentially promising role for VELscope was defined in a study of 20 consecutive patients undergoing surgical excision for previously diagnosed oral SCC.[68] The results showed the ability of the VELscope to detect areas of decreased autofluorescence in clinically normal-appearing tissue surrounding an established oral SCC (up to 2.5 cm beyond visible margins). This finding was further substantiated through molecular analysis showing LOH (loss of heterozygosity) and mutations of critical cell-cycle regulatory genes in the visibly normal-appearing tissue surrounding the tumor. Further development and investigation of this device in well-designed clinical trials tied in with detection of molecular biomarkers are required to further define this device as an effective treatment planning tool. The evidence to support VELscope as a primary screening/diagnostic tool for oral precancer and cancer remains limited at this time. Nonetheless, VELscope could prove to be a valuable adjunct for planning the management of already diagnosed precancerous and frankly malignant oral lesions.

SUMMARY

This exploration of the contemporary approach to diagnosis of oral cancer and precancerous lesions produces several key points:

- Oral cancer (SCC) is a genetic disease that results from the accumulation of mutations in genes that are critical for maintaining physiologic control of the cell cycle. The genetic aberrations permit the affected cells to behave in an uncontrolled manner. Such rogue behavior affects all of the cells in the field. For this reason a diagnosis of precancer (epithelial dysplasia) or carcinoma mandates ongoing clinical follow-up for an indefinite period: long-term clinical vigilance remains the most effective means of detecting and intercepting recurrent and new primary disease.
- The known risk factors for oral premalignant lesions and SCC are tobacco and alcohol. A variety of intrinsic contributing factors (eg, genetic susceptibility, immune status, metabolic capability) are likely responsible for encouraging the carcinogenic process. There are likely other risk factors that have not yet been identified. However, it is important to recognize that intraoral SCC is not attributable to UV radiation or HPV infection.
- Precancerous oral lesions present themselves clinically at a late stage in the protracted evolutionary process of malignant transformation of the surface epithelium. Given that the process likely continues after excision of a known oral cancer or precancerous lesion, ongoing and unrelenting clinical observation at regular intervals is essential.

- Noninvasive cell sampling techniques (conventional cytology and cytobrush biopsy) remain less diagnostically useful than the gold-standard tissue biopsy because they do not yield specific diagnoses. Cytopathologic interpretation yields only 3 possible diagnoses: negative, atypical, and positive. Furthermore, abnormal cytologic diagnoses (epithelial atypia and dysplasia/carcinoma) require further investigation (ie, conventional tissue biopsy) to establish a specific diagnosis. Unless or until the available cytodiagnostic techniques can be enhanced by linking cytomorphology with methods for genetic analysis of sampled cells and identification of biomarkers that indicate critical mutations, cytologic methods must not be used as a substitute for conventional biopsy, especially when there is concern about cancer or precancer.
- Several technologies that rely on TA and tissue reflectance have been developed and made available to clinicians in recent years. They are intended as adjuncts for enhancing the clinician's ability to screen for oral cancer and precancerous lesions. However, these technologies have proved to be less reliable or effective than conventional unaided oral examination performed by a trained clinician. Nonetheless, with further development these technologies could have potential applications as aids in treatment planning for management of previously diagnosed dysplastic lesions and SCCs.

REFERENCES

1. Horner MJ, Ries LAG, Krapcho M, et al. SEER Cancer Statistics Review, 1975–2006. National Cancer Institute, Bethesda (MD). Available at: http://seer.cancer.gov/csr/1975_2006. Accessed January, 2010.
2. Moore SR, Johnson NW, Pierce AM, et al. The epidemiology of tongue cancer: a review of global incidence. Oral Dis 2000;6(2):75–84.
3. Moore SR, Johnson NW, Pierce AM, et al. The epidemiology of mouth cancer: a review of global incidence. Oral Dis 2000;6(2):65–74.
4. Bishop JM. Molecular themes in oncogenesis. Cell 1991;64(2):235–48.
5. Hanahan D, Weinberg RA. The hallmarks of cancer. Cell 2000;100(1):57–70.
6. Funk GF, Karnell LH, Robinson RA, et al. Presentation, treatment, and outcome of oral cavity cancer: a National Cancer Data Base report. Head Neck 2002;24(2):165–80.
7. Canto MT, Devesa SS. Oral cavity and pharynx cancer incidence rates in the United States, 1975–1998. Oral Oncol 2002;38(6):610–7.
8. Mashberg A, Meyers H. Anatomical site and size of 222 early asymptomatic oral squamous cell carcinomas: a continuing prospective study of oral cancer. II. Cancer 1976;37:2149–57.
9. Moore C, Catlin D. Anatomic origins and locations of oral cancer. Am J Surg 1967;114:510–3.
10. Scully C, Bedi R. Ethnicity and oral cancer. Lancet Oncol 2000;1:37–42.
11. Rao DN, Ganesh B, Rao RS, et al. Risk assessment of tobacco, alcohol and diet in oral cancer–a case control study. Int J Cancer 1994;58:469–73.
12. Merchant A, Husain SSM, Hosain M, et al. Paan without tobacco: an independent risk factor for oral cancer. Int J Cancer 2000;86:128–31.
13. Brandwein-Gensler M, Hille JJ. Behind the cover: the gutkha story. Arch Otolaryngol Head Neck Surg 2003;129:699–700.
14. Lingen M. Head and neck. In: Kumar V, Abbas AK, Fausto N, editors. Robbins and Cotran pathologic basis of disease, professional edition. 8th edition. Philadelphia: Saunders, Elsevier; 2009. p. 744–9.

15. Califano J, van der Riet P, Westra W, et al. Genetic progression model for head and neck cancer: implications for field cancerization. Cancer Res 1996;56:2488–92.

16. Lippman SM, Hong WK. Molecular markers of the risk of oral cancer. N Engl J Med 2001;344:1323–6.

17. Blot WJ, McLaughlin JK, Winn DM, et al. Smoking and drinking in relation to oral and pharyngeal cancer. Cancer Res 1988;48:3282–7.

18. Wynder EL, Bross IJ, Feldman RM. A study of the etiological factors in cancer of the mouth. Cancer 1957;10:1300–23.

19. Hammond EC, Horn D. Smoking and death rates – report on forty-four months of follow-up of 187,783 men. JAMA 1958;166:1294–308.

20. Morse DE, Katz RV, Pendrys DG, et al. Smoking and drinking in relation to oral epithelial dysplasia. Cancer Epidemiol Biomarkers Prev 1996;5(10):769–77.

21. Brunnemann KD, Prokopczyk B, Djordjevic MV, et al. Formation and analysis of tobacco-specific N-nitrosamines. Crit Rev Toxicol 1996;26:121–37.

22. Hoffman D, Hoffman I. The changing cigarette, 1950–1995. J Toxicol Environ Health 1997;50:307–64.

23. Scully C, Bagan JV. Oral squamous cell carcinoma: overview of current understanding of etiopathogenesis and clinical implications. Oral Dis 2009;15:388–99.

24. Schecht NF, Franco EL, Pintos J, et al. Effect of smoking cessation and tobacco type on the risk of cancers of the upper aerodigestive tract in Brazil. Epidemiology 1999;10:412–8.

25. Baker F, Ainsworth SR, Dye JT, et al. Health risks associated with cigar smoking. JAMA 2000;284:735–40.

26. Shimkada R, Peabody JW. Tobacco control in India. Bull World Health Organ 2003;81:48–52.

27. Schildt EB, Eriksson M, Hardell I, et al. Oral snuff, smoking habits and alcohol consumption in relation to oral cancer in a Swedish case-control study. Int J Cancer 1998;77:341–6.

28. Lewin F, Norell SE, Johansson H, et al. Smoking tobacco, oral snuff and alcohol in the etiology of squamous cell carcinoma of the head and neck: a population-based case-referent study in Sweden. Cancer 1998;82:1367–75.

29. Marwick C. Increasing use of chewing tobacco, especially among younger persons, alarms surgeon general. JAMA 1993;269:195.

30. Winn DM, Blot WJ, Shy CM, et al. Snuff dipping and oral cancer among women in the southern United States. N Engl J Med 1981;304:745–9.

31. Idris AM, Ibrahim SO, Vasstrand EN, et al. The Swedish snus and the Sudanese toombak: are they different? Oral Oncol 1998;34:558–66.

32. Mashberg A, Garfinkel L, Harris S. Alcohol as a primary risk factor in oral squamous cell carcinoma. CA Cancer J Clin 1981;31:146–55.

33. Franceschi S, Levi F, La Vecchia C, et al. Comparison of the effect of smoking and alcohol drinking between oral and pharyngeal cancer. Int J Cancer 1999;83:1–4.

34. Hashibe M, Brennan P, Benhamou S, et al. Alcohol drinking in never users of tobacco, cigarette smoking in never drinkers, and the risk of head and neck cancer: pooled analysis in the International Head and Neck Consortium. J Natl Cancer Inst 2007;99(10):777–89.

35. Campisi G, Giovannelli L. Controversies surrounding human papilloma virus infection, head & neck vs oral cancer, implications for prophylaxis and treatment. Head Neck Oncol 2009;1(1):1–8.

36. Gillison ML, Koch WM, Capone RB, et al. Evidence for a causal association between human papillomavirus and a subset of head and neck cancers. J Natl Cancer Inst 2000;92:709–20.

37. Syrjanen S. HPV infections and tonsillar carcinoma. J Clin Pathol 2004;57:449–55.
38. Maitland NJ, Cox MF, Lynas C, et al. Detection of human papillomavirus DNA in biopsies of human oral tissue. Br J Cancer 1987;56:245–50.
39. Koch WM, Lango M, Sewell D, et al. Head and neck cancer in nonsmokers: a distinct clinical and molecular entity. Laryngoscope 1999;109:1544–51.
40. Lingen MW, Chang KW, McMurray SJ, et al. Overexpression of p53 in squamous cell carcinoma of the tongue in young patients with no known risk factors is not associated with mutations in exon 5–9. Head Neck 2000;22:328–35.
41. Sturgis EM, Wei Q. Genetic susceptibility – molecular epidemiology of head and neck cancer. Curr Opin Oncol 2002;14:310–7.
42. Tharp ME II, Shidnia H. Radiotherapy of verrucous carcinoma of the head and neck. Laryngoscope 1995;105:391–6.
43. Jyothirmayi R, Sankaranarayanan R, Varghese C, et al. Radiotherapy in the treatment of verrucous carcinoma of the oral cavity. Oral Oncol 1997;33(2):124–8.
44. Huang SH, Lockwood G, Irish J, et al. Truths and myths about radiotherapy for verrucous carcinoma of larynx. Int J Radiat Oncol Biol Phys 2009;73(4):1110–5.
45. Lippman SM, Hong WK. Second malignant tumors in head and neck squamous cell carcinoma: the overshadowing threat for patients with early-stage disease. Int J Radiat Oncol Biol Phys 1989;17(3):691–4.
46. Chi AC. Epithelial pathology. In: Neville BW, Damm DD, Allen CM, Bouquot JE, editors. Oral and maxillofacial pathology. 3rd edition. St. Louis (MO): Saunders Elsevier; 2009. p. 422–3.
47. Slaughter DP, Southwick HW, Smejkal W. Field cancerization in oral stratified squamous epithelium: clinical implications of multicentric origin. Cancer 1953; 6:963–8.
48. Axell T, Pindborg JJ, Smith CJ, et al. Oral white lesions with special reference to precancerous and tobacco-related lesions: conclusions of an international symposium held in Uppsala, Sweden May 18–21 1994. International Collaborative Group on Oral White Lesions. J Oral Pathol Med 1996;25:49–54.
49. "Leukoplakia", "keratosis", and intraepithelial squamous cell carcinoma of the head and neck. In: Batsakis JG, editor. Tumors of the head and neck: clinical and pathological considerations. Baltimore (MD): Williams & Wilkins; 1974. p. 121–9.
50. Pindborg JJ. Oral cancer and precancer. Bristol (UK): John Wright; 1980.
51. Crissman JD. Upper aerodigestive tract. In: Henson DE, Albores-Saavedra J, editors. 2nd edition. Pathology of incipient neoplasia, vol. 28. Philadelphia: WB Saunders; 1993. p. 44–63.
52. Hansen LS, Olson JA, Silverman SJR. Proliferative verrucous leukoplakia. A long-term study of thirty patients. Oral Surg Oral Med Oral Pathol 1985;60(3):285–98.
53. Morton TH, Cabay RJ, Epstein JB. Proliferative verrucous leukoplakia and its progression to oral carcinoma: report of three cases. J Oral Pathol Med 2007; 36(5):315–8.
54. Bagan JV, Jimenez Y, Sanchis JM, et al. Proliferative verrucous leukoplakia: high incidence of gingival squamous cell carcinoma. J Oral Pathol Med 2003;32(7): 379–82.
55. Cabay RJ, Morton TH Jr, Epstein JB. Proliferative verrucous leukoplakia and its progression to oral carcinoma: a review of the literature. J Oral Pathol Med 2007;36(5):255–61.
56. Campisi G, Giovannelli L, Ammatuna P, et al. Proliferative verrucous vs. conventional leukoplakia: no significantly increased risk of HPV infection. Oral Oncol 2004;40(8):835–40.

57. Bagan JV, Jimenez Y, Murillo J, et al. Lack of association between proliferative verrucous leukoplakia and human papilloma virus infection. J Oral Maxillofac Surg 2007;65(1):46–9.
58. Krutchkoff DJ, Eisenberg E, Anderson C. Dysplasia of oral mucosa: a unified approach to proper evaluation. Mod Pathol 1991;4:113–9.
59. Thomson PJ. Field change and oral cancer: new evidence for widespread carcinogenesis? Int J Oral Maxillofac Surg 2002;31(3):262–6.
60. Sciubba JJ. Improving detection of precancerous and cancerous oral lesions. Computer assisted analysis of the oral brush biopsy. U.S. Collaborative Oral CDx Study Group. J Am Dent Assoc 1999;130:1445–57.
61. Lingen MW, Kalmar JR, Karrison T, et al. Critical evaluation of diagnostic aids for the detection of oral cancer. Oral Oncol 2008;44:10–22.
62. Svirsky JA, Burns JC, Carpenter WM, et al. Comparison of computer-assisted brush biopsy results with follow-up scalpel biopsy and histology. Gen Dent 2002;50:500–3.
63. Sceifele C, Schmidt-Westhausen AM, Dietrich T, et al. The sensitivity and specificity of the Oral CDx technique: evaluation of 103 cases. Oral Oncol 2004;40: 824–8.
64. Poate TW, Buchanan JA, Hodgson TA, et al. An audit of the efficacy of oral brush biopsy technique in a specialist Oral Medicine unit. Oral Oncol 2004;40:829–34.
65. Patton LL, Epstein JB, Kerr AR. Adjunctive techniques for oral cancer examination and lesion diagnosis. A systematic review of the literature. J Am Dent Assoc 2008;139:896–905.
66. Gray MGL, Burls A, Elley K. The clinical effectiveness of toluidine blue dye as an adjunct to oral cancer screening in general dental practice. A West Midlands Development and Evaluation Service Report. 2000. Available at: http://www.pcpoh.bham. ac.uk/publichealth/wmhtac/pdf/toluidine_blue.pdf. Accessed January, 2010.
67. Huber MA, Bsoul SA, Terezhalmy GT. Acetic acid wash and chemiluminescent illumination as an adjunct to conventional oral soft tissue examination for the detection of dysplasia: a pilot study. Quintessence Int 2004;35:378–84.
68. Poh CF, Zhang L, Anderson DW, et al. Fluorescence visualization detection of field alterations in tumor margins of oral cancer patients. Clin Cancer Res 2006;12(22):6716–22.

Autoimmune Oral Mucosal Diseases: Clinical, Etiologic, Diagnostic, and Treatment Considerations

James J. Sciubba, DMD, PhD

KEYWORDS

• Oral mucosal diseases • Pemphigus vulgaris
• Mucosal pemphigoid • Oral lichen planus

Oral mucosal diseases are frequently encountered in daily practice, with associated degrees of concern and symptomatology on the part of the patient. Whereas most types of primary mucous membrane disease or conditions are commonplace, self-limiting, and episodic—such as recurrent aphthous stomatitis—others often may be difficult to characterize and manage, leading to longer than acceptable periods of discomfort and concern.

The autoimmune-associated diseases are a group of conditions that, although relatively uncommon, may lead to long periods of failed intervention, based on absence of a definitive diagnosis on one hand and unfamiliarity with effective therapeutics on the other. Involvement of areas beyond the oral cavity also may be a factor in overall disease management. The mouth is often the indicator or harbinger of more widespread lesions, with a corresponding opportunity to intervene early, leading to the opportunity for timely consultation with other members of the health care team, and the possible reduction of overall morbidity from these conditions.

Specific conditions discussed in this article include the classic autoimmune diseases pemphigus vulgaris (PV) (benign mucous membrane pemphigoid) and mucosal pemphigoid (MP) (cicatricial pemphigoid); as well as oral lichen planus (OLP), generally considered of autoimmune origin or, at a minimum, immune system mediated in the absence of a defined "lichen planus (LP) antigen."

The Milton J. Dance Head & Neck Center, The Greater Baltimore Medical Center, 6569 North Charles Street, Baltimore, MD 21204, USA
E-mail address: jsciubba@gbmc.org

Dent Clin N Am 55 (2011) 89–103
doi:10.1016/j.cden.2010.08.008
0011-8532/11/$ – see front matter © 2011 Elsevier Inc. All rights reserved.

PV

PV represents one of several mucocutaneous blistering diseases where oral lesions are commonly observed. It is considered a very rare condition in which an acantholytic process characterizes the skin and oral mucosal lesions. At times the oral lesions may dominate the initial presentation, with one recent study indicating that the oral mucosa is the primary site of 75% of new cases.[1] As is often the case for PV flaccid vesicles involving the keratinized and nonkeratinized lining, structures rapidly evolve into erosions and ulcerations with ill-defined margins and sloughing of the superficial layers of epithelium. The course of this condition is typically chronic and, before the introduction and use of systemic corticosteroids, was often fatal with death usually due to infection, sepsis, or dehydration.

A significant number of cases demonstrate a strong genetic or familial, as well as ethnic relationship, primarily within the Ashkenazi Jewish population and those of Mediterranean descent.[2,3] In common clinical practice within a multicultural and multi-racial setting, many groups are represented with classic PV. This is amplified when studying PV associations with HLA class II alleles (those entities largely responsible for T-lymphocyte recognition of desmogleins [Dsg] 3 peptides) and the country of origin of those studies.[4] In a large retrospective analysis of 159 cases a female/male ratio was approximately 2:1, while the mean age was 53 years.[4]

Cause or Pathophysiology

The pathologic process is mediated by autoantibodies that target the extracellular adhesion components, chiefly within the cadherin group of cell-cell adhesion mole-cules, particularly Dsg, which in the case of oral PV is mainly Dsg 3 and, to a much lesser extent, Dsg 1. Those individuals with predominantly or exclusively oral lesions only will demonstrate only antibodies to Dsg 3 in the early phases of this disease. However, if untreated, over time the phenomenon of epitope spread may occur with Dsg 1 recognized and attacked as well, producing concomitant skin lesions.[5,6] These components essentially anchor one epithelial cell to another above the basal cell layer. Resulting from this autoimmune attack is an intraepithelial separation immediately above the intact basal layer of cells that remains adherent to the underlying basement membrane zone (BMZ). More recently Cirillo and Prime[7] used a systems biology approach in studying keratinocyte and desmosomal interactions. In their model the adaptor protein, plakophylin 3 is a crucial molecule in mediating the cell-to-cell detachment or dysadhesion induced by PV IgG. The identification of a noncadherin desmosomal protein, *perp*, which, following PV autoantibody perturbation at the desmosome, is internalized, leading to a deficiency within the desmosome that, in turn, heightens the degradative effects on keratinocytes at their attachment sites.[8] Additionally, the possible role for antibodies directed against the 9 alpha nicotinic acetaldehyde receptor has been reviewed with a possible role for therapeutic alterna-tives concerning the addition of cholinergic agonists.[9] An apparent event in the path-ogenesis of desmosomal loss is that, subsequent to PV IgG attack at the desmosome, there is Dsg 3 endocytosis, followed by a corresponding retraction of keratin filaments toward the keratinocyte nucleus, followed by cell-cell adhesion compromise or loss, and that Dsg 3 internalization is intimately associated with the pathogenic activity of PV IgG activity.[10,11]

Drug-induced pemphigus may occur uncommonly. Drug classes involved include thiol group agents or those with a sulfhydryl radical (chiefly captopril and other ACE inhibitors) and penicillamine; as well as non-thiol medications, including rifampin, diclofenac, and phenol-containing drugs.[12]

Clinical Findings

Pemphigus may be seen across a wide age spectrum, though childhood onset is an uncommon event. Most cases are noted to occur in middle-aged to elderly adults. Onset is usually insidious, often masquerading as nonspecific ulcerations that heal within a few weeks with new lesions appearing elsewhere. Lesions are characterized as very short-lived vesicles initially and later, if untreated, bullae. Subsequent to vesicle rupture, tender and painful erosions and ulceration ensue. Palatal, buccal, and labial mucosal sites are favored, though no particular intraoral site is immune from involvement in untreated cases. Gingival involvement is often desquamative or erosive in nature. Oropharyngeal and hypopharyngeal involvement is characterized by odynophagia and hoarseness. Newly ruptured lesions will demonstrate a retracted surface epithelial component immediately adjacent to tender erosions and ulcerations (**Fig. 1**).

A rare form of pemphigus is paraneoplastic pemphigus, which, as the term implies, is associated with an underlying neoplastic condition, chiefly lymphoreticular in nature, though sarcomas may also be seen as the underlying neoplasm.[13] Lesions may develop before, coincident with, or following the diagnosis of neoplasia. With this condition there is almost always involvement of the labial vermilion surface and skin. Other mucosal sites involved beyond the oral cavity include the trachea and larynx.

Diagnosis

The diagnosis of PV involves routine as well as specific studies designed to characterize tissue alterations as well as to identify pathogenic antibodies, usually in patient tissue obtained by routine mucosal tissue biopsy (**Table 1**). The necessary step of immunologic verification involves use of a direct immunofluorescence technique in which the patient's mucosal specimen is paired with labeled or tagged immunoglobulin. Verification of diagnosis or quantification of the degree of antibody concentration or titer is available as indirect immunofluorescence (IIF); patient serum is proportionately diluted and reacted with nonpatient substrate tissue and labeled antihuman immunoglobulin.

Consideration of the precise site of tissue acquisition is important. Owing to the very friable nature of the oral mucosa in PV and the propensity of the mucosal surface to tear or simply shear away from the surgical blade, it is preferable to sample an area of mucosa that is not obviously involved with PV, but rather at a short distance from clinically evident disease. Therefore, perilesional tissue should be sampled.

Subsequent to obtaining a representative specimen, it must be managed carefully as to preserve the surface integrity. Additionally, the tissue must be placed into 10% neutral buffered formalin, as is routine for standard pathologic assessment, and also must be immersed in Michel's transport medium or buffer for direct immunofluorescence testing, as formalin-fixed tissue will not preserve the specimen properly for this technique.

The classic diagnostic light microscopic features of PV include a cleavage or separation of the suprabasal layer of the surface epithelium with the basal layer of cells remaining adherent to the basement region. This layer of cells assumes a so-called "tombstone" quality, while free-floating, acantholytic cells above the basal layer (Tzanck cells) are seen secondary to desmosomal loss and corresponding tonofilament retraction **Fig. 2**.

In addition to routine microscopy, direct immunofluorescence (DIF) studies will demonstrate the presence of IgG antibody and activated complement (C-3) along the cell surface within the intercellular space **Fig. 2C**. Similarly, IIF studies using the

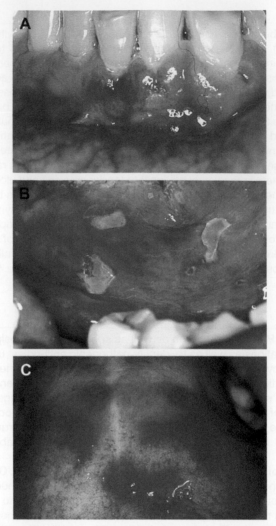

Fig. 1. PV: (*A*) Collapsed vesicles and superficial ulcerations over the attached gingiva. (*B*) Anterior floor of the mouth showing scattered collapsed vesicles. (*C*) Widespread painful and tender palatal ulcerations.

| Table 1 | |
Clinical differential diagnosis of PV	
MP	Allergic or hypersensitivity reaction
Erosive lichen planus	Lupus erythematosus
Erythema multiforme	Epidermolysis bullosa
Viral infection	—

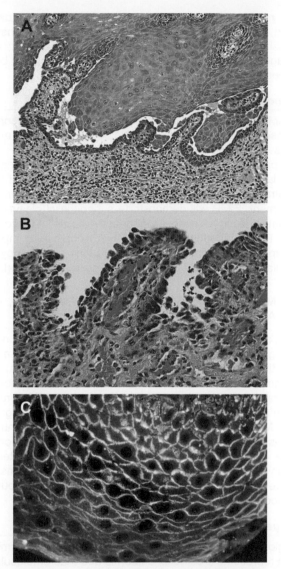

Fig. 2. PV: (*A*) Characteristic suprabasal separation or cleavage of the stratified squamous epithelium obtained from an intact perilesional area. (*B*) Free unattached squamous cells are present within the separation. Note the uniformly adherent and intact basal cell layer. (*C*) Direct immunofluorescence specimen demonstrating labeled anti-human IgG within the intercellular space, the site of host antibody directed at Dsg 3, the pemphigus antigen, within the oral epithelium.

patient's serum, though less sensitive than DIF, may be used to demonstrate the presence of serum or circulating antibody levels.

An alternative to direct immunofluorescence to demonstrate the presence of intercellular IgG antibodies is through the use of an immunoperoxidase staining technique where the primary antibody is tagged with the peroxidase enzyme that subsequently catalyzes activation of a chromogen at the site of antigen-antibody binding in tissue.

In addition to routine IIF, circulating antibody may also be demonstrated by an enzyme-linked immunosorbent assay (ELISA) where great sensitivity has been shown in establishing the diagnosis and response to treatment; although it has been cautioned against as there has been some lack of correlation between disease activity and antibody levels.[14,15]

Differential Diagnosis

Loss of surface epithelial integrity will also be noted in other conditions that might be similar to PV. These include MP, paraneoplastic pemphigus (PNP), and a rare subset of PV: pemphigus vegetans (Pveg).

In Pveg, skin is predominantly involved with labial vermilion border and oral mucosal lesions, followed later in the course of the disease by an epithelial hyperplasia with corresponding intraepithelial aggregates of large numbers of eosinophils, IgG, and activated complement.[16] MP will demonstrate subepithelial cleavage with IgG and activated complement along the epithelial-connective tissue interface, with the epithelial surface intact. PNP is immunologically and microscopically complex with subepithelial and intraepithelial separations seen on routine microscopy, while a large number of epithelial and basement membrane antigens are targeted.

MP: MUCOUS MEMBRANE PEMPHIGOID, CICATRICIAL PEMPHIGOID, AND BENIGN MUCOUS MEMBRANE PEMPHIGOID

MP represents an additional chronic blistering disease of autoimmune origin, without a particular inciting or triggering stimulus. Clinical involvement may extend to the eye or ocular conjunctival mucosa, or may remain restricted to the oral cavity, with oral disease usually antedating the onset of ocular involvement. A recent study noted a 37% incidence rate of developing ocular disease in cases where oral disease developed initially, with a mean interval of 19.3 months between the diagnosis or oral MP and ocular MP.[17] MP is a member of a group or family of autoimmune subepithelial blistering diseases that includes bullous pemphigoid (BP), gestational pemphigoid, linear IgA disease, epidermolysis bullosa acquisita, and bullous systemic lupus erythematosus; though oral mucosal involvement with those conditions beyond MP is uncommon to rare. MP is considered to be generally heterogeneous in nature with several autoantibodies identified as pathogenic.

Cause and Pathogenesis

The anatomic region of the oral mucosa that is directly affected in terms of cause is the BMZ. This region represents a complex anatomic and macromolecular continuum of proteins derived from the keratinocyte and fibroblast populations of cells that form a functional network of fibrillar proteins and glycoproteins that enable a stable association of surface epithelium and underlying lamina propria and submucosa, across the basement membrane complex. MP represents one such disease state where there is a perturbation of this macromolecular complex by an autoimmune process. As with many autoimmune conditions, the initial or triggering event in producing the disease is unknown, though some drugs may have a role in this process, as is the case with PV. Autoantibodies in MP are predominantly directed against BP 180 and less commonly against laminin 5 (epiligrin), type 7 collagen, or the $\beta4$ subunit of $\alpha6\beta4$ integrin (a transmembrane keratinocyte-specific integrin), and the a6 integrin subunit.[18] IgG and C3 deposits are usually identified in the basement membrane complex or hemidesmosomes with immunofluorescence techniques, where many distinct antigenic components have been identified overall.[19–21]

The actual mechanisms of epithelial separation or dysadhesion from the lamina propria may occur in a variety of ways. Subsequent to the binding of autoantibodies to target antigens within the BMZ complement, activation follows with release of chemoattractants and subsequent recruitment of eosinophils and neutrophils. Proteolysis follows, along with further release of chemoattractants and cytokines, with ultimate focal tissue damage and epithelial-subepithelial dysadhesion. A second mechanism by which the same tissue effect will evolve is by direct interference with the function of adhesion of BP 180, laminin 5 (epiligrin), or integrins (chiefly α6β4). There is a secondary disassembly of hemidesmosomes resulting in defective adhesion and separation. Finally, there may be a resultant defect in cell signaling followed by disturbed hemidesmosome assembly and induction of proinflammatory cytokines contributing to epithelial-subepithelial separation or dysadhesion.[22]

Clinical Findings

MP may arise initially at any mucosal site, including oral and conjunctival mucosa most commonly, but also the external genitalia, anus, and upper gastrointestinal tract or esophagus.[23] Of note, however, is that 85% of cases will have oral involvement without concomitant skin involvement, and it may be the only site of disease.

Lesions distribution will chiefly involve the gingiva, palatal mucosa, and buccal mucosa; and less over the tongue, alveolar ridges and lips (**Fig. 3**A–C). The gingival presentation is typically one of painful erythematous and tender erosions with desquamation, either spontaneously or with very minimal physical trauma, such as with tooth brushing. Often there is an inability to maintain oral care with consequent heavy accumulation of plaque and an additional inflammatory burden from this source. Small vesicles may be observed that rupture easily, but, in comparison to those of PV, are

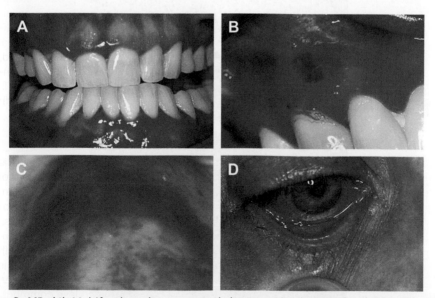

Fig. 3. MP: (*A*) Multifocal erythematous and desquamative lesions distributed over the attached gingiva, with wide areas of ulceration extending onto the alveolar gingival mucosa. (*B*) A slightly irregular blood-filled vesicle over the attached gingiva. (*C*) Ruptured vesicles, erosions, and ulcerations along the hard and soft palatal junction. (*D*) Early ocular involvement by mucosal, pemphigoid with intense inflammation and tiny vesicles toward the outer canthus.

longer-lasting and more well-defined. With rupture of vesicles, tender erosions result along with functional discomfort. Over time, there may be scarring (cicatrization) at sites of repeated vesiculo-erosive lesion development and healing, chiefly over the posterior soft palate, uvula, tonsillar folds, ventral tongue, and floor of the mouth.

Establishment of this diagnosis is often in the dental office, given the frequency of initial oral mucosal presentation. Subsequent to diagnosis and in association with initial treatment of oral lesions, patients must be evaluated by an ophthalmologist, as conjunctival involvement is common and may result in corneal damage and possible blindness if untreated **Fig. 3**D. In cases where pharyngeal involvement is present, an evaluation with a gastroenterologist is indicated. Additionally, in cases where there may be epistaxis, nasal crusting, and mucosal adhesions, an otolaryngologist must be consulted.

Diagnosis

Routine microscopic evaluation of either an intact vesicle or perilesional tissue will signal the presence of a clear subepithelial separation in the absence of acantholysis, as the site of antigen-antibody interaction is below the basal epithelial layer **Fig. 4**A. Absence of basal cell adhesion to the lamina propria will be noted, as will a monocellular inflammatory infiltrate with lymphocytes and plasma cells in evidence. Ultrastructural examination, although not a routine study, will show a separation within the lamina lucida.

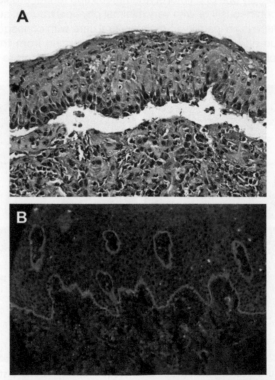

Fig. 4. MP: (*A*) Perilesional mucosa demonstrates a cleavage plane along the epithelial basement membrane region. No basal cells remain adherent to the lamina propria. (*B*) Direct immunofluorescence microscopy of an intact area of attached gingiva adjacent to active MP shows the characteristic deposition of IgG in a smooth linear pattern along the basement membrane region.

Key to the establishment of the diagnosis of MP and its separation from other vesiculo-erosive conditions is the performance of direct immunofluorescence microscopy, where the patient's mucosal tissue is treated with fluorescein-labeled antihuman immunoglobulin for demonstration of in vivo-bound immunoglobulin. Most cases (up to 90%) will show the presence of IgG or C3 in a smooth and linear pattern along the basement membrane **Fig. 4**B. Less commonly, there may be linear deposits of IgA and IgM in the same pattern.

Other studies to demonstrate the pathognomonic features of MP, although not routine, include immunoelectron microscopy, as well as immunochemical modalities involving immunoprecipitation and immunoblotting. High sensitivity and specificity in searching for circulating autoantibodies are possible with the use of recombinant proteins, such as BP 180, by ELISA testing.

The use of laser canning confocal microscopy has been advocated recently for diagnostic distinction among subepithelial blistering diseases by way of detecting the presence and precise location of in vivo-bound immunoglobulin within the patient's tissue.[24]

Differential Diagnosis

Distinguishing MP from other subepithelial blistering and erosive diseases that may involve mucosa where there may be immune deposits along the basement membrane region may prove difficult. The wide spectrum of autoimmune blistering diseases that can manifest within the area of the basement membrane include BP, linear IgA disease, and epidermolysis bullosa acquisita. In the oral cavity in particular, MP must be chiefly separated from PV and erosive LP. The presence of scarring may help separate MP from these; however, in the early phases of the disease, scarring may not be easily seen or present.

LP

OLP may occur independent of or in concert with cutaneous lesions, either in a synchronous or metachronous fashion. It is almost always seen to affect stratified squamous epithelium only. It is relatively uncommon, of unknown cause, with oral mucosal lesions persisting far longer than cutaneous lesions. Oral mucosal lesions and, to a lesser degree, genital lesions may be severe and often painfully debilitating. It is distributed worldwide, with women affected more commonly than men, with lesions arising mostly within the fifth to sixth decades.

This disease affects from 1% to 2% of the general adult population and is the most common disease of noninfectious origin in oral medicine or oral pathology practices.[25]

Cause and Pathogenesis

The specific cause of OLP is unknown, but is known to be mediated by a T-cell–mediated chronic inflammatory process. The antigen or altered protein responsible for the immune system driving this disease is unknown, though the antigen may be a self-peptide, thus defining LP as an autoimmune condition. Sugerman and colleagues[26] state that an early pathogenic event might involve the unmasking or expression of a keratinocyte-derived antigen at the site of a future lesion that may be induced by systemic drugs, contact allergens, physical trauma, viral or bacterial infection, or an as yet unidentified entity. The result is T-cell recognition of the LP antigen followed by a complex set of events resulting in local apoptosis of keratinocytes. These events may involve many antigen specific events or mechanisms, including antigen presentation by lesional keratinocytes, activation of CD-4$^+$ and CD-8$^+$ cells, clonal expansion of antigen-specific T-cells, and keratinocyte death by antigen-specific cytotoxic CD-8+ T-cells. This proposed mechanism is highly theoretical and, in part, controversial, though the cause of OLP must be considered complex and multifactorial with immune cell dysfunction being central in association with cytokine expression, including tumor necrosis factor-a, interleukins, and upregulation of matrix metalloproteinases and p53, with ultimate keratinocyte death.[27] Men and women are affected in nearly equal numbers, with children rarely affected. Stress may be a modulating factor but is not thought to represent a primary cause. There is no convincing relationship between diabetes mellitus or hypertension as once proposed, though a more likely relationship to these diseases and LP may be an associated lichenoid drug reaction as it relates to their management. A possible relationship to hepatitis C in some geographic areas may exist, however. This has been proposed in certain Italian patients with the HLA-DR6 class II allele, but not in British patients.[28]

Clinical Findings

A wide spectrum of mucosal alterations is noted with reticular, atrophic, erosive, papular, and, occasionally, bullous lesions. Sites of involvement most commonly are the buccal mucosa, gingiva, tongue, and vermilion portion of the lips, though any intraoral site can be affected. Several clinical forms or types of LP have been described within the oral cavity, with the reticular form being the most common and most easily recognized type (**Fig. 5**A). This form is characterized by the presence of numerous interlacing and branching white lines or striae that, in aggregate, produce annular or lacy configurations, most commonly over the buccal mucosa bilaterally.

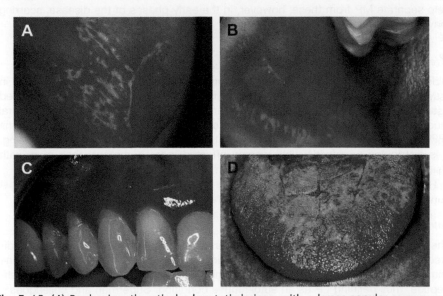

Fig. 5. LP: (A) Predominantly reticular keratotic lesions, with a lesser papular component cover much of the buccal mucosa, with similar lesions over the opposite buccal mucosa. (B) Well-defined erosive or ulcerative LP is surrounded by a linear reticular keratotic component. The base of the ulcerated area is covered with a firmly-adherent fibrinous component with a sharp border against the intact lichenoid periphery. (C) Attached gingival involvement by LP is characterized by atrophic, erythematous, edematous, and tender qualities in the absence of vesicles or ulceration. (D) The dorsum of the tongue with uniformly keratinized features further defined by keratotic plaques and concomitant papillary atrophy.

It also is commonly seen over the dorsal aspect of the tongue and less commonly over the attached gingiva and vermilion portion of the lips. Papular areas of keratinization may also be seen in concert with striae or may rarely be a predominant clinical presentation, though uncommonly so within the oral cavity.

Erosive LP will show central areas of ulceration with a well-defined periphery and a fibrinous or pseudomembranous base that is firmly adherent to the submucosa (**Fig. 5C**). Sites most commonly involved with this form of LP are the buccal mucosa and, less so, the lateral tongue region labial vermilion border (**Fig. 5B**).

The atrophic form of LP presents as erythematous lesions with a thinned, glassy surface appearance that may, on occasion, also be noted to possess very fine, peripheral white striae (**Fig. 5C**). These forms may present uniformly, but will often be combined with reticular and plaque types of presentation. Affected most commonly with this variant is the attached gingiva, which may be desquamative in nature, tender, friable, and easily bleeding over multiple sites in all quadrants with variable degrees of severity, which will often compromise routine hygiene measures, thus contributing to symptoms.

The plaque form of OLP is characteristically seen over the dorsum of the tongue, with resemblance to leukoplakia, though with a multifocal and more widespread distribution (**Fig. 5D**). The plaques are smooth and generally flat, but may be slightly elevated. This form may also be noted over areas of the buccal mucosa, particularly toward the inner aspect of the labial commissures.

Oral lichenoid lesions may present in a similar clinical and histologic fashion to idiopathic LP, but will have a definable cause. Most commonly, a drug-related cause can be identified, as well as sensitivity to certain dental materials. Additionally, the oral mucosal lesions of chronic graft-versus-host disease will show similarity; however, oral lichenoid lesions will tend to be less often symmetric and unilateral, and more likely to be erosive than idiopathic disease.[29]

Differential Diagnosis

To be included in the clinical separation of LP from other conditions is lupus erythematosus, hypersensitivity to dental materials and lichenoid drug reactions, graft-versus-host disease, MP, and leukoplakia.

Diagnosis

Incisional biopsy of nonulcerated, involved mucosa is generally sufficient to establish a working diagnosis. In routinely prepared specimens a typical subepithelial band of lymphocytes will be present that parallel the surface with extension of lymphocytic infiltration or "trafficking" into the overlying epithelium. The epithelial basal layer will often be overrun and, in areas, obliterated with cell separation and vacuolation, basement membrane pooling or laking effect, and loss or apoptosis of keratinocytes seen with formation of colloid or Civatte bodies representing individually necrotic keratinocytes within the basal layer region. On occasion there will be a "sawtooth pattern" of epithelial ridges seen, while at the free surface, hyperkeratosis will be present (**Fig. 6A–C**). Absence of dysplasia is the rule. Recent studies attempting to identify higher risk cases for possible malignant transformation have identified two biomarkers, podoplanin and ABCG2, as candidates.[30]

In cases of diagnostic difficulty, direct immunofluorescence studies will demonstrate the presence of fibrinogen along the BMZ in a shaggy pattern, unlike that seen in other autoimmune diseases where immunoglobulin and complement deposition are present (**Fig. 6D**).

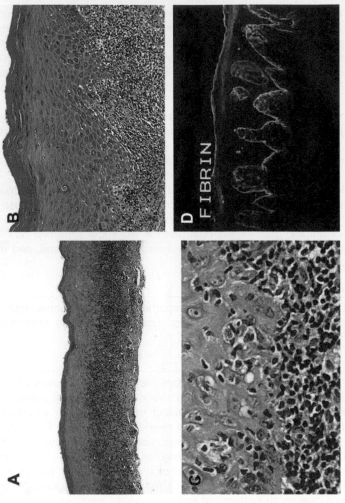

Fig. 6. LP: (*A*) A low-power view demonstrates the characteristic dense, band-like chronic inflammatory cell infiltrate along the basement membrane region, with an intact overlying epithelial layer. (*B*) Obliteration or obfuscation of the basal layer in areas with a moderate degree of intercellular edema. (*C*) Intraepithelial infiltration that is predominantly lymphocytic in nature is present, with loss of a definitive basal layer of cells. (*D*) Direct immunofluorescence of an intact area of reticular LP demonstrates the deposition of fibrin along the BMZ in a shaggy, ill-defined pattern, which extends into the lamina propria.

Comments on Approaches to Treatment

Fundamental to a successful clinical therapeutic outcome of the discussed diseases is management of the overall autoimmune and immune-mediated inflammatory pathology inherently characteristic to them as a whole. Immune system management for the conditions detailed here ranges from simple observation, as in the case of asymptomatic reticular LP to significant systemic immunosuppression with nearly all cases of PV. Intermediate levels of treatment intervention in cases of erosive and ulcerative LP and MP may involve early and temporary systemic immunosuppression in the acute management phase, followed by long-term control measures, chiefly using topical therapies of immunosuppression and possibly local antimicrobial strategies. Topical management may at times be augmented by local intralesional corticosteroid placement in areas that are incompletely controlled.

In cases of PV, systemic treatment typically will involve corticosteroids, initially up to 1 mg per kg, in concert with initiation of steroid-sparing methodologies and supportive measures. In addition, a topical corticosteroid component may be considered as a possible systemic steroid-sparing technique as well. Following achievement of control, consideration will be given to a gradual tapering dose of systemic steroid within a consolidation phase, which will be facilitated by the then established steroid-sparing effect of earlier prescribed drugs that might include azathioprine, mycophenolate mofetil, dapsone, and others. In cases where a combined approach is unsuccessful, intravenous administration of immune globulin G (IvIg) might be employed; whereas the most severe of cases could involve the use of plasmapheresis and cyclophosphamide therapy. Needless to say, the management at this level must involve the patient's primary care physician and specialty members of the health care team with input from the dental provider.

Following establishment of an acceptable treatment response, long-term follow-up is necessary. Maintenance of treatment results may be life-long with regard to PV and MP. LP follow-up may also be over considerable periods of time.

SUMMARY

Autoimmune diseases involving the oral mucosa are not limited to those presented and discussed here. Others conditions of this type also include the oral presentation of lupus erythematosus, certain forms of epidermolysis bullosa and linear IgA disease. As management of these diseases progresses, continued advances in molecular pathogenesis will allow insight into which strategies can employed in interfering with the complex cascade of events leading to mucosal impairment and clinical morbidity. Currently, the use of the chimeric monoclonal antibody rituximab for recalcitrant PV has proven to be remarkably effective.[31,32] The mechanism of action in this case is quite specific in comparison to treatments to date where several immune system components are suppressed. In cases where rituximab treatment is used, there is a demonstrable depletion of B-lymphocytes as well as a decrease in desmoglein-specific T cells.[33]

REFERENCES

1. Ishii N, Maeyama Y, Karashima T, et al. A clinical study of patients with pemphigus vulgaris and pemphigus foliaceous: an 11-year retrospective study (1996–2006). Clin Exp Dermatol 2008;33(5):641–3.
2. Kircheli D, David M, Frusic-Zlotkin M, et al. The distribution of pemphigus vulgaris Ig subclasses and their reactivity with desmoglein 3 and 1 in pemphigus patients and their first-degree relatives. Br J Dermatol 2000;143:337–42.

3. Mignogna MD, Fortuna G, Leuci C. Oral pemphigus. Minerva Stomatol 2009; 58(10):501–18.
4. Ahmed AR, Wagner R, Khatri K, et al. Major histocompatibility complex haplotypes and class II genes in non-Jewish patients with pemphigus vulgaris. Proc Natl Acad Sci U S A 1991;88:5056–60.
5. Harman KE, Seed PT, Gratian MJ, et al. The severity of cutaneous and oral pemphigus is related to desmoglein 1 and 3 antibody levels. Br J Dermatol 2001;144:775–80.
6. Endo H, Rees TD, Hallmon WW, et al. Disease progression from mucosal to mucocutaneous involvement in a patient with desquamative gingivitis associated with pemphigus vulgaris. J Periodontol 2008;79(2):369–75.
7. Cirillo N, Prime SS. Desmosomal interactome in keratinocytes: a systems biology approach leading to an understanding of the pathogenesis of skin diseases. Cell Mol Life Sci 2009;66(21):3517–33.
8. Nguyen B, Dusek RL, Beaudry VG, et al. Loss of desmosomal protein perp enhances the phenotypic effects of pemphigus vulgaris autoantibodies. J Invest Dermatol 2009;129(7):1710–8.
9. Femiano F. Pemphigus vulgaris: recent advances in our understanding of its pathogenesis. Minerva Stomatol 2007;56(4):215–23.
10. Calkins CC, Setzer SV, Jennings JM, et al. Desmoglein endocytosis and desmosome disassembly are coordinated responses to pemphigus autoantibodies. J Biol Chem 2006;281(11):7623–34.
11. Delva E, Jennings JM, Calkins CC, et al. Pemphigus vulgaris IgG-induced desmoglein 3 endocytosis and desmosomal disassembly are mediated by a clathrin- and dynamin-independent mechanism. J Biol Chem 2008;283:18303–13.
12. Scully C, Challacombe SJ. Pemphigus vulgaris: update on etiopathogenesis, oral manifestations and management. Crit Rev Oral Biol Med 2002;13(5):397–408.
13. Anhalt GJ, Kim SC, Stanley JR, et al. Paraneoplastic pemphigus: an autoimmune mucocutaneous disease associated with neoplasia. N Engl J Med 1990;323:1729–35.
14. Belloni-Fortina A, Faggion D, Pigozzi B, et al. Detection of autoantibodies against recombinant desmoglein 1 and 3 molecules in patients with pemphigus vulgaris: correlation with disease extent at the time of diagnosis and during follow-up. Clin Dev Immunol Volume 2009. DOI:10.1155/2009/187864.
15. Huang CH, Chen CC, Wang CJ, et al. Using desmoglein 1 and 3 enzyme-linked immunosorbent assay as an adjunct diagnostic tool for pemphigus. J Chin Med Assoc 2007;70(2):65–70.
16. Markopoulos AK, Antoniades DZ, Zaraboukas T. Pemphigus vegetans of the oral cavity. Int J Dermatol 2006;45(4):425–8.
17. Higgins GT, Allan RB, Hall R, et al. Development of ocular disease in patients with mucous membrane pemphigoid involving the oral mucosa. Br J Ophthalmol 2006;90(8):964–7.
18. Bhol KC, Goss L, Kumari S, et al. Antibodies to human alpha 6 integrin in patients with oral pemphigoid. J Dent Res 2001;80(8):1711–5.
19. Bhol KC, Colon JE, Ahmed AR. Autoantibody in mucous membrane pemphigoid binds to an intracellular epitope on human β4 integrin and causes basement membrane zone separation in oral mucosa in an organ culture model. J Invest Dermatol 2003;120(4):701–2.
20. Uitto J, Pulkkinen L. Molecular complexity of the cutaneous basement membrane zone. Mol Biol Rep 1996;23(1):35–46.
21. Chan L. Human skin basement membrane in health and in autoimmune disease. Front Biosci 1997;2:d343–52.

22. Bedane C, McMillan J, Balding S, et al. Bullous pemphigoid and cicatricial pemphigoid autoantibodies react with ultrastructurally separable epitopes on the BP 180 ectodomain: evidence that BP 180 spans the lamina lucida. J Invest Dermatol 1997;108:901–7.
23. Fleming TE, Korman NJ. Cicatricial pemphigoid. J Am Acad Dermatol 2000;43: 571–91.
24. Wozniak K, Kazama T, Kowlaewski C. A practical technique for differentiation of subepidermal bullous diseases. Arch Dermatol 2003;139:1007–11.
25. Bowers KE, Sexton J, Sugerman PB. Commentary. Clin Dermatol 2000;18:497–8.
26. Sugerman PB, Savage NW, Walsh LJ, et al. The pathogenesis of oral lichen planus. Crit Rev Oral Biol Med 2002;13(4):350–65.
27. Scully C, Carrozzo M. Oral mucosal disease: lichen planus. Br J Oral Maxillofac Surg 2008;46:15–21.
28. Carrozzo M, Brancatello F, Dametto E, et al. Hepatitis C virus-associated oral lichen planus: is the geographical heterogeneity related to HLA-DR6? J Oral Pathol Med 2005;34:204–8.
29. Nakamura S, Hiroki A, Shinohara M, et al. Oral involvement in chronic graft-versus-host disease after allogeneic bone marrow transplantation. Oral Surg Oral Med Oral Pathol Oral Radiol Endod 1996;82:556–63.
30. Shi P, Liu W, He QB, et al. Podoplanin and ABCG2: malignant transformation risk markers for oral lichen planus. Cancer Epidemiol Biomarkers Prev 2010;19: 844–9.
31. Cianchini G, Corona R, Frezzolini A, et al. Treatment of severe pemphigus with rituximab: report of 12 cases and a review of the literature. Arch Dermatol 2007;143(8):1033–8.
32. Joly P, Roujeau JC, D'Incan M, et al. A single cycle of rituximab for the treatment of severe pemphigus. N Engl J Med 2007;357(6):545–52.
33. Zambruno G, Borradori L. Rituximab immunotherapy in pemphigus: therapeutic effects beyond B-cell depletion. J Invest Dermatol 2008;128(12):2745–57.

Differential Diagnosis of Temporomandibular Disorders and Other Orofacial Pain Disorders

Jeffrey P. Okeson, DMD[a],*, Reny de Leeuw, DDS, PhD[b]

KEYWORDS

• Temporomandibular disorders
• Temporomandibular joint disorders • Neuropathic pain
• Migraine • Tension type headache

The focus of this article is on the differential diagnosis of pain disorders that typically fall outside the realm of dental diseases. There are a great variety of such conditions— too many to review here. Therefore, this article discusses the differential diagnosis of a few of the more common orofacial pain conditions the dentist may face in a practice. These conditions are divided into two sections: temporomandibular disorders (TMD) and other common orofacial pain disorders. The first section reviews common TMD that are the responsibility of the dentist to identify and manage. The second section reviews some common orofacial pain disorders that the dentist needs to recognize but for which the dentist may not be the primary care provider.

TMD

TMD is a collective term that includes a number of clinical complaints involving the muscles of mastication, the temporomandibular joint (TMJ), or associated orofacial structures.[1] TMD are a major cause of nondental pain in the orofacial region and are considered a subclassification of musculoskeletal disorders. In many TMD patients the most common complaint originates from the muscles of mastication rather than from the TMJ. Therefore, the terms TMJ dysfunction or TMJ disorder are inappropriate for many complaints arising from the masticatory structures. It is

[a] Department of Oral Health Science, Division of Orofacial Pain, D-142, College of Dentistry, University of Kentucky, 800 Rose Street, Lexington, KY 40536-0297, USA
[b] Division of Orofacial Pain, D-530, College of Dentistry, University of Kentucky, 800 Rose Street, Lexington, KY 40536-0297, USA
* Corresponding author.
E-mail address: okeson@uky.edu

Dent Clin N Am 55 (2011) 105–120
doi:10.1016/j.cden.2010.08.007
0011-8532/11/$ – see front matter © 2011 Elsevier Inc. All rights reserved.

for this reason that the American Dental Association adopted the term "temporomandibular disorder."[2]

Signs and symptoms associated with TMD are a common source of chronic pain complaints in the head and orofacial structures. These complaints can be associated with some generalized musculoskeletal problems and even somatization, anxiety, and depression. The primary signs and symptoms associated with TMD originate from the masticatory structures and, therefore, are associated with jaw function. Patients often report pain in the preauricular areas, face, or temples. Reports of pain during mouth opening or chewing are common. Some individuals may even report difficulty speaking or singing. TMJ sounds are also frequent complaints and maybe described as clicking, popping, grating, or crepitus. In many instances, the joint sounds are not accompanied by pain or dysfunction, and are merely a nuisance to the patient. However, on occasion, joint sounds may be associated with locking of the jaw during opening or closing, or with pain. Patients may even report a sudden change in their bite coincident with the onset of the painful condition.

It is important to appreciate that pain associated with most TMD is increased with jaw function. Because this is a condition of the musculoskeletal structures, function of these structures generally increases the pain. When a patient's pain complaint is not influenced by jaw function, other sources of (orofacial) pain should be suspected.

TMD can be subdivided into two broad categories related to their primary source of pain and dysfunction: masticatory muscle disorders and intracapsular (TMJ) disorders. A description of the most common disorders in each category is reviewed below. A more complete review of TMD can be found elsewhere.[3]

Masticatory Muscle Disorders

Definition
Functional disorders of masticatory muscles are probably the most common TMD complaint of patients seeking treatment in the dental office. With regard to pain, they are second only to odontalgia (ie, tooth or periodontal pain) in terms of frequency. They are generally grouped in a large category known as masticatory muscle disorders.

Clinical features
The two major symptoms of functional TMD problems are pain and dysfunction. Certainly the most common complaint of patients with masticatory muscle disorders is muscle pain, which may range from slight tenderness to extreme discomfort. Pain felt in muscle tissue is called myalgia. The pain is commonly described in terms such as dull, achy, or tender. The symptoms are often associated with a feeling of muscle fatigue and tightness. Patients will usually describe the location of the pain as broad or diffuse, and the pain is often bilateral. This complaint is quite different than the specific location reported in intracapsular disorders.

The severity of muscle pain is generally directly related to the amount of functional activity. Therefore, patients often report that the pain affects their ability to open their mouth, chew, and speak. If the patient does not report an increase in pain associated with jaw function, the disorder is not likely related to a masticatory muscle problem and other diagnoses should be considered.

The clinician should appreciate that not all muscle pain is the same.[3] Some patients suffer with relatively simple overuse muscle pain called "local muscle soreness." Clinically, the local muscle soreness manifests as tenderness or pain on palpation. Other patients may experience a more regional muscle condition such as myofascial pain. Clinically, myofascial pain is characterized by the presence of localized, firm, hypersensitive bands of muscle tissue called trigger points.[4] These areas create a source of deep pain input that can lead to central excitatory effects resulting in pain referral. This condition manifests as pain on palpation with referral of pain in the surrounding or remote tissues. Sometimes these remote tissues can be teeth, and the primary complaint that the patient may have is tooth pain. It is important that the dentist realizes that the site of pain is not always the same as the source of the pain. In this hypothetical case of myofascial pain, there is nothing wrong with the teeth (the site of the pain); however, it would be easy for the dentist to miss the correct diagnosis if the muscles of mastication (the source of the pain) were not included in the diagnostic work-up. It is also important to realize that myofascial pain originating from cervical muscles may refer pain into the orofacial region. Treating the site of pain in these instances would not result in improvement of the symptoms.

Dysfunction is a common clinical symptom associated with masticatory muscle disorders. Clinically, this may be seen as a decrease in the range of mandibular movement. When muscle tissues have been compromised by overuse, any contraction or stretching increases the pain.[5] Therefore, to maintain comfort, the patient restricts movement within a range that does not increase pain. The restriction may be at any degree of opening depending on where discomfort is felt. The restriction may also be partly due to contraction of the antagonistic muscles, a phenomenon that is called protective cocontraction. In many myalgic disorders the patient is able to slowly open wider but this increases the pain.

Acute malocclusion is another condition that is often associated with masticatory muscle pain. Acute malocclusion refers to any sudden change in the occlusal position that has been created by a disorder. An acute malocclusion may result from a sudden change in the resting length of a muscle that controls jaw position. When this occurs the patient describes a change in the occlusal contacts of the teeth. The mandibular position and resultant alteration in occlusal relationships depend on the muscles involved. For example, the malocclusion associated with slight functional shortening of the inferior lateral pterygoid is clinically evident as disclusion of the posterior teeth on the ipsilateral side and premature contact of the anterior teeth (especially the canines) on the contralateral side. With functional shortening of the elevator muscles (clinically a less detectable acute malocclusion), the patient will generally complain of a sensation of heavier tooth contact on the ipsilateral side. It is important to realize that an acute malocclusion is the result of the muscle disorder and not the cause. Therefore, treatment should never be directed toward correcting the malocclusion by means of occlusal adjustments. Rather, it should be aimed at eliminating the muscle disorder. When the muscle disorder is resolved, the occlusal condition will return to normal.

Etiologic considerations

Myalgia can arise from a number of different causes. The most common cause is an increased level of muscle use. Although the exact origin of this type of muscle pain is debated, some investigators suggest it is related to vasoconstriction of the relevant nutrient arteries and the accumulation of metabolic waste products in the muscle tissues.[5] Within the ischemic area of the muscle certain algogenic substances (eg, bradykinins, prostaglandins) are released, causing muscle pain.

Increased muscle use maybe the result of activities that are outside the normal functional activities of chewing, swallowing, and speaking. Such activities are considered parafunctional and these activities are more likely to compromise the muscle tissues and create pain. Activities such as daytime clenching of the teeth or sleep-related bruxing are common parafunctions that may lead to muscle pain.[6] In addition to clenching and bruxing, habits such as chewing gum and biting lips, cheeks, and finger nails are also considered to be parafunctional activities. It should be appreciated that these activities are very common and do not lead to pain in most individuals.

A misunderstood but very important concept for the clinician to appreciate is the fact that masticatory muscle pain is not strongly correlated with increased muscle activity such as in spasm.[7-9] In fact, studies reveal that the resting activity of the masticatory muscles as measured by electromyography of patients with chronic muscle pain is no different than that of asymptomatic controls. Therefore the majority of masticatory muscle pain patients are not experiencing spasms.

It is now appreciated that muscle pain can be influenced and actually initiated by the central nervous system through antidromic effects leading to neurogenic inflammation in the peripheral structures. When these peripheral structures are muscles, this is clinically felt as muscle pain. This type of muscle pain is referred to as "centrally mediated myalgia" and can be a difficult problem to manage for the dentist since the peripheral structures, such as teeth, jaw, and muscles are not the significant cause of the pain. In these instances, the central mechanisms need to be addressed, which cannot be accomplished by classic dental therapies. Owing to the involvement of central mechanisms, increased levels of emotional stress and other sources of deep pain may likely influence masticatory muscle pain disorders.[10]

Management considerations
A detailed description of the management of each of the conditions is not the goal of this article and, therefore, other sources should be consulted. However, because some simple behavior modifications may reduce parafunctional use of the muscles, a few first-tier management options are described in this section. Making the patient aware that his or her maxillary and mandibular teeth should not be touching each other except to speak, chew, or swallow is an important first step. In addition, for most masticatory muscle conditions, soft diet, rest, moist heat, and (possibly) nonsteroidal anti-inflammatory drugs (NSAIDS) are usually helpful. Teaching the patient to keep the teeth apart and the mouth relaxed when the jaw is not used is very beneficial if not crucial in reducing pain.[11] If sleep-related bruxism is suspected, a stabilization appliance may be helpful.

TMJ

Definition
The signs associated with functional disorders of the TMJ are probably the most common findings when examining a patient for masticatory dysfunction. Many of these signs do not produce painful symptoms and, therefore, the patient may not seek treatment. When present, however, they generally fall into three broad categories: derangements of the condyle-disc complex, structural incompatibility of the articular surfaces, and inflammatory joint disorders. The first two categories have been collectively referred to as disc-interference disorders. The term disc-interference disorder was first introduced by Welden Bell[12] to describe a category of functional disorders that arises from problems with the condyle-disc complex. Some of these problems are due to a derangement or alteration of the attachment of the disc to the condyle; others to an incompatibility between the articular surfaces of the condyle, disc, and fossa; still others to the fact that relatively normal structures have been extended beyond their normal range of movement. With time, inflammatory disorders can arise from a localized response of the TMJ tissues to loading or trauma. These disorders are often the result of chronic or progressive disc derangement disorders.

Clinical features
The two major symptoms of functional TMJ problems are pain and dysfunction. Joint pain can arise from healthy joint structures that are mechanically abused during

function, from impingement of tissues, or from structures that have become inflamed. Pain originating from healthy structures or impingements is felt as sharp, sudden, and (sometimes) intense pain that is closely associated with joint movement. When the joint is rested, the pain resolves instantly. The patient often reports the pain as being localized to the preauricular area. If the joint structures have become inflamed, the pain is reported as constantly dull or throbbing, even at rest, yet accentuated by joint movement.

Dysfunction is common with functional disorders of the TMJ. Usually it presents as a disruption of the normal condyle-disc movement often with the production of joint sounds. The joint sounds may be a single event of short duration known as a click. If this is loud, it may be referred to as a pop. Crepitation is a multiple, rough, gravel-like sound described as grating or grinding. Dysfunction of the TMJ may also present as catching sensations when the mouth is opened. Sometimes the jaw can actually lock. Dysfunction of the TMJ is always directly related to jaw movement.

A single click during opening of the mouth is often associated with an anterior displaced disc that is returned to a more normal position during the opening movement. This condition is referred to as a "disc displacement with reduction."[3] Often when the patient closes the mouth a second click is felt which represents the re-displacement of the disc to the anterior displaced position (**Fig. 1**). This single opening click associated with disc displacement with reduction should be fairly repeatable. When the patient reports a single, loud, popping or cracking sound that cannot be easily repeated, the clinician should think about the possibility of an adherence.[13] An adherence can occur as a result of prolonged static loading of the joint. In such a case, the lubrication is squeezed out of the contacting joint surfaces and this causes the surfaces stick together. On opening, this union can be disrupted and normal mouth opening resumes.

For some patients the disc displacement progresses and the disc may not be able to return to its normal relationship with the condyle during opening. This condition is referred to as a "disc displacement without reduction."[3] When this occurs, the patient often cannot open fully because the disc is blocking the translation of the condyle. For this reason the condition is often referred to as a "closed lock" (**Fig. 2**). Additional clinical characteristics include a deflection to the ipsilateral side on opening and protrusion, and restriction of movement to the contralateral side due to the limited ability of the condyle to translate.

Crepitation is usually related to roughness of the articular surfaces because of remodeling or osteoarthritis. Typically this is found in patients who have experienced a disc displacement without reduction or in whom radiographically notable bony changes are present. It can also be a sign of perforation of the disc or the retrodiscal tissues. If crepitation is the only symptom or sign a patient presents with, treatment is not usually indicated. Likewise, if the patient presents with a painless clicking TMJ that does not affect the quality of life, treatment is not indicated. However, the patient should be reassured and educated with regard to the origin of the sounds and, if indicated, instructed to avoid parafunctional activities.

Etiologic considerations
The cause of intracapsular disorders of the TMJ is most commonly related to trauma.[14-16] This trauma may manifest itself as either macrotrauma or microtrauma. In cases of macrotrauma a single blow to the mandible can lead to a disruption of the normal biomechanical functions of TMJ. The traumatic event typically injures joint structures—elongating ligaments or damaging articular surfaces. Once ligaments have been elongated their biomechanical function is changed—often creating instability of the joint. This could eventually lead to disc displacement. Instability and

A Normal Disc Position   **B** Disc Displacement

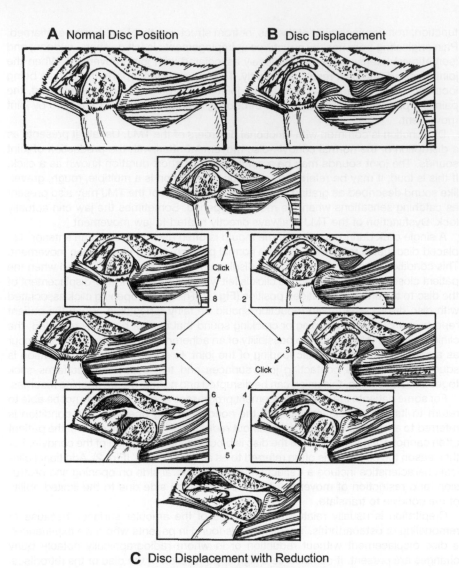

C Disc Displacement with Reduction

Fig. 1. (*A*) Normal condyle-disc relationship. (*B*) Disc displacement. (*C*) The movement of the condyle with a disc displacement. Note the clicking between 3 and 4, and again between 8 and 1. (*Adapted from* Okeson JP. Management of temporomandibular disorder and occlusion. 6th edition. St Louis (MO): CV Mosby; 2008. p. 181; with permission.)

disc displacement may both cause abnormal or unfavorable loading in the TMJ, and this may lead to osteoarthritic changes.[17]

Microtrauma, a small amount of loading force repeated over a long period of time, may lead to changes in joint structures. When the teeth are brought into heavy contact and the joint structures are loaded, there is a momentary reduction of blood flow in the small capillaries that supply the joint structures, resulting in hypoxia (a reduced supply of oxygen). Under circumstances of hypoxia, the metabolism of the local cell populations may alter. The byproducts of the altered metabolism may form free radicals when oxygen becomes available again, once the load on the tissues is reduced and the

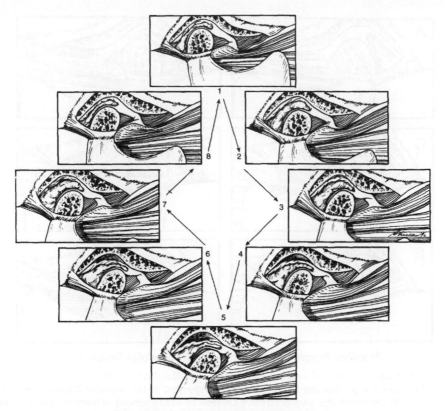

Disc Displacement without Reduction

Fig. 2. The movement of the condyle with a disc displacement without reduction. Note the disc is constantly maintained in the dislocated position (a closed lock). (*Adapted from* Okeson JP. Management of temporomandibular disorder and occlusion. 6th edition. St Louis (MO): CV Mosby; 2008. p. 185; with permission.)

capillaries are reperfused. Free radicals may also be generated by direct mechanical trauma and tissue damage. Free radicals are very unstable molecules with a strong affinity for electrons. If these electrons are taken from adjacent healthy tissues, the integrity of these tissues can be compromised. This process is known as a "hypoxia-reperfusion injury."[13,18] The subtle changes that may occur could consist of a decrease in the lubrication quality of the synovial fluid creating more friction during joint movement. It may also affect the articular surfaces of the joint creating a softening of this tissue called "chondromalacia." The compromised lubrication and softening of articular surfaces can cause the disc to displace from its normal position between the condyle and fossa.

Once the disc is displaced, joint loading can occur on nonarticular surfaces such as the retrodiscal tissue behind the disc. Because these tissues are highly vascularized and well innervated, compression often leads to pain. With further loading these tissues can breakdown allowing the condyle to directly load the articular fossa. Continued loading of these structures can result in loss of the articular surface of the condyle and fossa. The end result of this breakdown is osteoarthritis or degenerative joint disease (**Fig. 3**).

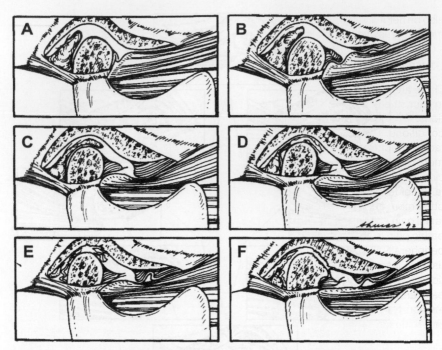

Possible Progressive Stages of Intracapsular Disorders

Fig. 3. The various states of internal derangement of the TMJ. (*A*) Normal joint. (*B*) Slight disc displacement. (*C*) Disc displacement. (*D*) Impingement of the retrodiscal tissues. (*E*) Retrodiscitis. (*F*) Osteoarthritis. (*Adapted from* Okeson JP. Management of temporomandibular disorder and occlusion. 6th edition. St Louis (MO): CV Mosby; 2008. p. 197; with permission.)

Management considerations

As previously mentioned, a detailed description of the management of each of the conditions is not the goal of this article and, therefore, other sources should be consulted.[3] However, because some simple behavior modifications may reduce the loading of the joints, a few first-tier management options are described in this section. Because comparative studies have shown that conservative therapies provide similar results to the more aggressive ones, the general rule should always be to provide the most conservative therapy first.

The principle concept for managing most intracapsular disorders is to reduce loading of the joint structures so that remodeling and adaptation of the involved structures can take place.[17] It is important to note that for adaptation to take place and for normal function to return, it is not necessary to restore the disc position. The patient needs to know that, if loading can be controlled, intracapsular disorders are often self limiting. Teaching the patient to reduce loading by simple approaches such as a softer diet with slower chewing can be very helpful. The patient should be instructed to avoid nonfunctional tooth contacts, such as clenching the teeth, chewing gum, and other oral parafunctional activity such as biting the fingernails or a pencil. If nighttime bruxism is suspected, a stabilization appliance may be considered for sleep-related bruxism. In cases of a painful disc displacement with reduction, an anterior positioning appliance may be useful, but care should be taken to use this appliance only during sleep, as longer use such as during the day and night may result in malocclusion. Clock-regulated NSAIDs may also be helpful. Only after these types of therapies fail to control the patient's pain should more aggressive therapies be considered (eg, arthrocentesis or arthroscopy).

OTHER COMMON OROFACIAL PAIN DISORDERS

There are many conditions that manifest painful symptoms in the orofacial structures. In fact, there are many textbooks that have been devoted solely to these conditions.[19,20] However, it is not the goal of this article to elaborate on all orofacial pain conditions. The reader merely needs to appreciate that the scope of pain in the orofacial structures is multifaceted and complex. This article highlights a few of the more common types of orofacial pain disorders that should be recognized by the clinician so that patients may receive the most appropriate care. Many of these conditions fall outside the normal realm of the dental practice and, therefore, should be referred to other more appropriate health care providers. This article discusses four common orofacial pain conditions. The first two conditions are neuropathic pain conditions. Neuropathic pain is a painful condition that has its origin within the neural tissue itself, either peripherally or centrally. With neuropathic pain there is nothing wrong with the somatic tissues; instead, the problem lies in how the nervous system is transmitting information to the sensory cortex. Neuropathic pain is divided into episodic neuropathic pain and continuous neuropathic pain disorders. The next two are migraine and tension-type headache. These conditions are considered primary headaches by the International Headache Society.[21]

Episodic Neuropathic Pains

Definition
As described earlier, pains that arise from abnormalities in the neural structures are called "neuropathic pains." Episodic neuropathic pains are characterized by a quick off-and-on pattern of pain.

Clinical features
Episodic neuropathic pains are characterized by periods of very brief, but intense, electrical shock-like pain followed by total remission. Usually, the individual is able to localize the site of pain quite well. The site, however, does not identify the correct source, because many are projected heterotopic pains. The term paroxysmal neuralgia has been used to describe this electrical shock-like pain. The most common is trigeminal neuralgia. Trigeminal neuralgia is characterized by a bright, stimulating, electric shock-like-quality pain that radiates into one of the three branches of the trigeminal nerve. The maxillary branch is affected most often, followed by the mandibular branch. The ophthalmic branch is affected the least often. The pain is extremely intense, usually lasting only a few seconds. On occasion it may last minutes, but this is rare. The pain is typically brought on by innocuous stimuli such as touching the face, shaving, or brushing the teeth. Between episodes the individual is usually pain free; however, if the episodes are frequent, there may be a lingering, dull aching pain.[22] Other neuralgias are glossopharyngeal neuralgia, geniculate neuralgia, superior laryngeal neuralgia, and nervus intermedius neuralgia.[23]

Etiologic considerations
The most common cause of trigeminal neuralgia is thought to be related to a demyelinization of the nerve root as it exits the pons before reaching the foramen.[24] This demyelinization may be secondary to pressure applied to the nerve by either a vessel in the brain[25] or an intracranial tumor.[26] Systemic demyelinization disorders such as multiple sclerosis may also lead to symptoms indicative of trigeminal neuralgia.[27]

However, in the majority of cases, none such factors can be identified, which renders the cause unknown.

Management considerations

Management of trigeminal neuralgia begins initially with medications that attempt to stabilize the nerve membranes. The most effective medications are typically anticonvulsive medications such as carbamazepine and oxcarbazepine, even though these medications may have serious side effects.[28–30] Medications with less evidence of effectiveness but with a better side-effect profile include gabapentin[31] or pregabalin.[32] If medications do not adequately resolve the pain, there are several surgical options varying from peripheral procedures such as rhizotomy to central procedures, including microvascular decompression surgeries and gamma knife procedures that may be considered.[1]

Continuous Neuropathic Pains

Definition

Some neuropathic pains may have fluctuating intensities but never go away. These disorders are called continuous neuropathic pains and are currently some of the most difficult orofacial pain conditions to successfully manage.

Clinical features

Continuous neuropathic pains are characterized by a dull, yet burning, pain. The pain is ongoing and unremitting, yet the intensity can show patterns of fluctuation. The pain is often accompanied by other neurologic signs (ie, anesthesia, paresthesia, hypoesthesia, hyperesthesia). Although the pain is present in a particular location, there is no evidence of any tissue changes or disease. When this pain is felt in the region of the teeth it can be a difficult challenge for the dentist. The pain may have the same clinical characteristics of a true toothache, which makes the correct diagnosis challenging for the clinician. However, helpful hints to consider are the duration of the pain and the fact that stimulation of the site of neuropathic pain (ie, with hot or cold) does not typically influence the intensity of the pain.[33]

Etiologic considerations

The cause of continuous neuropathic pain is not well understood. Certainly, trauma to a peripheral nerve can result in deafferentation (ie, an ongoing pain condition).[34] However, some continuous neuropathic pains seem to spontaneously appear without any obvious cause. It is believed that the central nervous system can change (neuroplasticity) resulting in the processing of information that is not appropriate for the peripheral stimulus (central sensitization).

Management considerations

Management of continuous neuropathic pains is very difficult. Research is only beginning to help us understand the central mechanisms that seem to contribute to this painful condition. Medical management is the first line of treatment; however, the medications that are presently available do not consistently help all patients. At best, we can reduce pain and improve quality of life, but total elimination of this type of pain is very difficult. Sometimes the tricyclic antidepressants[35] such as amitriptyline or desipramine can be helpful. The anticonvulsive medications such as gabapentin or pregabalin may also be helpful.[31,32,36] Often a trial of some of these medications and others may be needed to determine the most effective treatment. It is important to remember that neuropathic pains typically do not respond to NSAIDs or opioids. A complete list of management options for continuous neuropathic pain can be found elsewhere.

Migraine

Definition

Migraine is a common, intense and debilitating headache. It is what the general public refers to whenever someone has a "really bad headache." It is a primary headache with central etiologies. The International Headache Society has two major designations for migraine: migraine with aura and migraine without aura.[37]

Clinical features

Migraine is characterized by throbbing, moderate-to-severe, often debilitating pain. Sixty percent of the time the headache is unilateral and often reported in the temple or behind the eye. Migraine can be felt in the maxillary arch, thus referred to as "midface migraine." This can be a diagnostic problem for the dental clinician because the pain can be felt in or around the teeth. The patient will often report nausea, photophobia, phonophobia, and osmophobia, and will seek a dark, quiet room. The pain is aggravated by routine physical activity and sometimes even simple head movements. The pain episodes may occur at any time of the day or night but most frequently occur on arising in the morning. The pain episode commonly lasts 4 to 72 hours in adults and 2 to 4 hours in children.[38] Scalp tenderness occurs in two-thirds of the patients during or after the headache.

Some migraine patients report a complex of focal neurologic symptoms that immediately precedes the headache.[39] This is called the "aura" and usually develops in 5 to 20 minutes and lasts less than 1 hour. When present, the aura is commonly characterized by visual, sensory, or motor phenomena, and may even include language and brainstem disturbances. The visual symptoms are the most common phenomena associated with aura. Visual symptoms can be characterized by sensations of flashes of light before the eyes (photopsia), the partial loss of sight (scotoma), or a zigzag, flashing colored phenomenon that migrates across the visual field (teichopsia). Sensory symptoms such as paresthesia[40] can occur. Motor effects may present as focal fatigue or difficulty with speech.

Etiologic considerations

Migraine affects approximately 12% of the population, with about 18% females and about 6% males being affected.[41] Migraine most often appears in the first 3 decades of life.

Studies suggest that migraine patients have a genetic susceptibility to this pain condition, with 50% to 60% of migraine patients having parents that also experience migraines.[42] Migraine is considered a neurovascular phenomenon because both neuralgic and vascular structures are involved in the pathophysiology. This system of neural innervation of the intracranial vessels is called the trigeminovascular system. Present evidence suggests that there is a neurologic trigger in the brainstem that initiates a cascade of events that result in neurogenic inflammation of the cranial vessels producing the headache.[43]

Management considerations

The management of migraine with or without aura involves patient education and pharmacologic approaches. Patients who experience migraine headaches need to understand basic information about their pain condition. They need to know that even though the pain is very severe, it is still benign. An important aspect of education is having the patient identify any triggering factors that initiate the migraine attack. Triggers may be initiated by exposures to certain foods, alcohol, odors, stress, or even changes in eating or sleeping patterns. The patient should be asked to maintain a pain diary which helps identify factors that are associated with the initiation of the headache. Once these factors are identified, efforts are made to avoid them so as to reduce the number of migraine attacks.

Pharmacologic management of migraine can be divided into two types: medications that are used to abort a migraine at its start and medications that are used to prevent migraine attacks. The choice of which management strategy to use is determined by the frequency of the migraine attacks. As a general rule, migraine attacks that are infrequent are managed with abortive medications so that treatment is immediately initiated during the onset of the attack. When migraine attacks occur so often that they significantly interfere with the patient's daily activities, preventive medications should be considered.[44] If abortive medications are used 2 days per week or more, the patient may develop rebound headache or medication-overuse headache.

A class of medications that has been proven helpful in aborting a migraine is the triptans, of which there are many.[44] These drugs seem to stop the neurogenic inflammation in the meningeal (dural) vasculature[45] and they may also act within the brain. Frequent migraines are best managed by prescribing daily medication so as to prevent them from occurring. Beta-adrenergic agents (beta blockers) such as propranolol or metoprolol[46] or calcium channel blockers such as nifedipine or verapamil[47] have proven effective. In addition, the tricyclic antidepressants have shown to be useful—especially amitriptyline.[44,48] Finally, anticonvulsants such as topiramate and divalproex sodium also have proven to be efficacious in the prevention of migraines.[49]

Dentists do not normally prescribe such medications unless they have advanced training in orofacial pain, oral medicine, or oral surgery because many of the drugs have significant side effects, especially on the cardiovascular system (eg, propranolol, sumatriptan). Although most are quite safe in a healthy patient, the medically compromised patient or chronic pain patient who uses other medications may experience significant problems that will need proper attention by appropriate health care professionals.

Tension-type Headache

Definition
Tension-type headache is a primary headache felt as a bilateral dull, aching pain usually felt in the shape of a tight band around the head. It is estimated that as many as 74% of the general population experience this type of headache at least once a year.[50]

Clinical features
Tension-type headache is the most common headache reported in the general population. The headache is described as a dull, nonpulsatile tightness, or pressure felt in the occipital, parietal, temporal, and frontal regions. In 90% of the cases, the pain is felt bilaterally.[50] Some will describe the feeling of a tight "headband" compressing their head as if they were wearing a tight cap. Most tension-type headaches are of mild or moderate intensity, rarely becoming debilitating as with migraine. Most tension-type headaches are episodic, lasting an average of 12 hours, although the duration can vary greatly (30 minutes to 72 hours).[51] Accompanying symptoms may consist of either photophobia or phonophobia but not both. Nausea is not associated with tension-type headache.[52]

Etiologic considerations
Although tension-type headache is the most common headache experienced by humans, its pathophysiology remains unclear. Part of the problem may be that tension-type headache likely has a central etiologic mechanism, especially involving

the limbic structures. Emotional stress, anxiety, and depression seem to present causal relationships with tension-type headaches.[53,54] However, there are many other disorders that result in headache that present with the same clinical characteristics of tension-type headache. For example, trigger points associated with myofascial pain (discussed previously) result in a headache at the referred site that is often clinically described by the patient as a tension-type headache. This type of headache is secondary to the myofascial condition and, therefore, should not be classified as a tension-type headache. Similarly, patients with sleep bruxism may awake with headache as a secondary symptom. Also morning headache in the temporal area is frequent associated with sleep respiratory disorders related to snoring or sleep apnea.[55,56] The headache should always be classified to the primary disorder, which will assist in selecting the proper treatment.

Management considerations
Like many pain disorders, management of tension-type headache begins with patient education. The sufferer needs to identify those factors that aggravate the condition as well as those that help relieve it. It is often helpful to have the patient maintain a headache diary so that factors that are not commonly considered be recognized. The patient should be encouraged to decrease intake of caffeine (coffee, tea, soft drinks) and alcohol, as well as any medications that have been chronically used for the headache (rebound headache). The patient should be informed that eliminating these substances may at first increase the frequency and intensity of the headaches. After 1 to 2 weeks, the withdrawal effects should subside.

Since emotional stress often plays an important role in tension-type headache, the patient should be assessed for any significant stressors and, if identified, corrective behaviors or avoidance should be encouraged. Stress management skills can be important therapies with tension-type headache. Relaxation training and biofeedback techniques[53,54] can also be very helpful. All these are frequently performed by a psychologist trained in cognitive-behavioral therapy. If a major depression disorder or anxiety disorder is present, these conditions need to be managed by the proper health care provider.

As with migraines, depending on the frequency of the headache, tension-type headaches are treated either with abortive or preventive medications. However, there are to date no evidence-based guidelines indicating which medications are most effective. To abort infrequent tension-type headaches, judicious use of mild analgesics (eg, aspirin, ibuprofen) may be needed, but the patient should be aware of the potential complications. NSAIDs are often helpful, especially if the patient has not been using them previously. If one NSAID is not effective, another should be tried. To prevent frequent tension-type headaches low dosages of a tricyclic antidepressant such as nortriptyline and amitriptyline can be helpful. They are best taken before bed time because of their sedative effects.

When the tension-type headache symptoms are secondary to another disorder, therapy needs to be extended to that disorder. For example, when the headache is associated with a masticatory muscle disorder, the muscle disorder needs to be managed.[3] Headache upon awaking may be related to nocturnal bruxism or sleep breathing disorders (apnea-hypopnea syndrome) and several approaches can be used to address this.

SUMMARY

There are many types of pain conditions that produce orofacial pain. The most common are dental and periodontal pains, which are highlighted elsewhere in this issue. Some of the other common pain disorders are musculoskeletal, which in the orofacial structures are called TMD. These disorders need to be identified by the dentist. In most cases they can be managed by relatively simple strategies. There are still many other pain disorders of the head and neck that are unrelated to the dental structures. The dentist should be able to differentiate these and refer the patient to the appropriate health care provider for appropriate care.

REFERENCES

1. De Leeuw R. Orofacial pain: guidelines for classification, assessment, and management. 4th edition. Chicago: Quintessence Publ. Co.; 2008.
2. Griffiths RH. Report of the President's Conference on Examination, Diagnosis and Management or Temporomandibular Disorders. J Am Dent Assoc 1983;106:75–7.
3. Okeson JP. Management of temporomandibular disorders and occlusion. 6th edition. St Louis (MO): The CV Mosby Company; 2008.
4. Simons DG, Travell JG, Simons LS, et al. Pain and dysfunction: a trigger point manual. 2nd edition. Baltimore (MD): Williams & Wilkins; 1999.
5. Mense S. The pathogenesis of muscle pain. Curr Pain Headache Rep 2003;7(6): 419–25.
6. Glaros AG, Burton E. Parafunctional clenching, pain, and effort in temporomandibular disorders. J Behav Med 2004;27(1):91–100.
7. Carlson CR, Okeson JP, Falace DA, et al. Comparison of psychologic and physiologic functioning between patients with masticatory muscle pain and matched controls. J Orofac Pain 1993;7:15–22.
8. Lund JP, Widmer CG. An evaluation of the use of surface electromyography in the diagnosis, documentation, and treatment of dental patients. J Craniomandib Disord 1988;3:125–37.
9. Klasser GD, Okeson JP. The clinical usefulness of surface electromyography in the diagnosis and treatment of temporomandibular disorders. J Am Dent Assoc 2006;137(6):763–71.
10. Okeson JP. Bell's orofacial pains. 6th edition. Chicago: Quintessence Publishing Co Inc; 2005. Chapter 595–104.
11. Carlson C, Bertrand P, Ehrlich A, et al. Physical self-regulation training for the management of temporomandibular disorders. J Orofac Pain 2001;15:47–55.
12. Bell WE. Temporomandibular joint disease. Dallas (TX): Egan Company; 1960.
13. Nitzan DW. 'Friction and adhesive forces'–possible underlying causes for temporomandibular joint internal derangement. Cells Tissues Organs 2003;174(1–2): 6–16.
14. Yun PY, Kim YK. The role of facial trauma as a possible etiologic factor in temporomandibular joint disorder. J Oral Maxillofac Surg 2005;63(11):1576–83.
15. Zhang ZK, Ma XC, Gao S, et al. Studies on contributing factors in temporomandibular disorders. Chin J Dent Res 1999;2(3–4):7–20.
16. Grushka M, Ching VW, Epstein JB, et al. Radiographic and clinical features of temporomandibular dysfunction in patients following indirect trauma: a retrospective study. Oral Surg Oral Med Oral Pathol Oral Radiol Endod 2007;104(6): 772–80.
17. Brandt KD, Dieppe P, Radin E. Etiopathogenesis of osteoarthritis. Med Clin North Am 2009;93(1):1–24, xv.
18. Milam SB, Zardeneta G, Schmitz JP. Oxidative stress and degenerative temporomandibular joint disease: a proposed hypothesis. J Oral Maxillofac Surg 1998; 56(2):214–23.

19. Olesen JGP, Ramandon N, Tfelt-Hansen P, et al. The headaches. 3rd edition. Philadelphia: Lippincott, Williams and Wilkins; 2006.
20. Dalessio DJ, Silberstein SD. Wolff's headache and other head pain. 6th edition. New York: Oxford University Press; 1993.
21. Olesen J. The international classification for headache disorders. Cephalalgia 2004;24(Suppl 1):1–160.
22. McArdle MJ. Atypical facial neuralgia. In: Hassler R, Walker AE, editors. Trigeminal neuralgia. Stuttgart (Germany): Georg Thieme Verlag; 1970. p. 35–42.
23. Okeson JP. Bell's orofacial pains. 5th edition. Chicago: Quintessence Publishing Co, Inc; 1995. Chapter 17. p.403–55.
24. Devor M, Amir R, Rappaport ZH. Pathophysiology of trigeminal neuralgia: the ignition hypothesis. Clin J Pain 2002;18(1):4–13.
25. Love S, Coakham HB. Trigeminal neuralgia: pathology and pathogenesis. Brain 2001;124(Pt 12):2347–60.
26. Celik SE, Kocaeli H, Cordan T, et al. Trigeminal neuralgia due to cerebellopontine angle lipoma. Case illustration. J Neurosurg 2000;92(5):889.
27. Fiske J, Griffiths J, Thompson S. Multiple sclerosis and oral care. Dent Update 2002;29(6):273–83.
28. Wiffen PJ, McQuay HJ, Moore RA. Carbamazepine for acute and chronic pain. Cochrane Database Syst Rev 2005;3:CD005451.
29. Gomez-Arguelles JM, Dorado R, Sepulveda JM, et al. Oxcarbazepine monotherapy in carbamazepine-unresponsive trigeminal neuralgia. J Clin Neurosci 2008; 15(5):516–9.
30. Nasreddine W, Beydoun A. Oxcarbazepine in neuropathic pain. Expert Opin Investig Drugs 2007;16(10):1615–25.
31. Gilron I, Bailey JM, Tu D, et al. Nortriptyline and gabapentin, alone and in combination for neuropathic pain: a double-blind, randomised controlled crossover trial. Lancet 2009;374(9697):1252–61.
32. van Seventer R, Feister HA, Young JP Jr, et al. Efficacy and tolerability of twice-daily pregabalin for treating pain and related sleep interference in postherpetic neuralgia: a 13-week, randomized trial. Curr Med Res Opin 2006; 22(2):375–84.
33. Graff-Radford SB, Solberg WK. Atypical odontalgia. J Craniomandib Disord 1992;6(4):260–5.
34. Fields HL, Rowbotham M, Baron R. Postherpetic neuralgia: irritable nociceptors and deafferentation. Neurobiol Dis 1998;5(4):209–27.
35. Haanpaa ML, Gourlay GK, Kent JL, et al. Treatment considerations for patients with neuropathic pain and other medical comorbidities. Mayo Clin Proc 2010; 85(3 Suppl):S15–25.
36. Jensen TS, Madsen CS, Finnerup NB. Pharmacology and treatment of neuropathic pains. Curr Opin Neurol 2009;22(5):467–74.
37. Oleson J, Tfelt-Hansen P, Welch KM. The headaches. 2nd edition. Philadelphia: Lippincott, Williams and Wilkins; 1999.
38. Lipton RB, Bigal ME, Steiner TJ, et al. Classification of primary headaches. Neurology 2004;63(3):427–35.
39. Stewart WF, Shechter A, Lipton RB. Migraine heterogeneity. Disability, pain intensity, and attack frequency and duration. Neurology 1994;44(6 Suppl 4):S24–39.
40. Russell MB, Olesen J. A nosographic analysis of the migraine aura in a general population. Brain 1996;119(Pt 2):355–61.
41. Lipton RB, Bigal ME, Diamond M, et al. Migraine prevalence, disease burden, and the need for preventive therapy. Neurology 2007;68(5):343–9.

42. Walters WE, Silberstein SD, Dalessio DJ. Inheritance and epidemiology of head-ache. In: Dalessio DJ, Silberstein SD, editors. Wolff's headache and other head pain. 6th edition. New York: Oxford University Press; 1993. p. 42–58.
43. Lambert GA, Zagami AS. The mode of action of migraine triggers: a hypothesis. Headache 2009;49(2):253–75.
44. Silberstein SD. Practice parameter: evidence-based guidelines for migraine headache (an evidence-based review): report of the Quality Standards Subcommittee of the American Academy of Neurology. Neurology 2000;55(6):754–62.
45. Williamson DJ, Hargreaves RJ. Neurogenic inflammation in the context of migraine. Microsc Res Tech 2001;53(3):167–78.
46. Diener H. Pharmacological approaches to migraine. J Neural Transm Suppl 2003; 64:35–63.
47. Adelman JU, Adelman RD. Current options for the prevention and treatment of migraine. Clin Ther 2001;23(6):772–88 [discussion: 71].
48. Bendtsen L, Jensen R. Amitriptyline reduces myofascial tenderness in patients with chronic tension-type headache. Cephalalgia 2000;20(6):603–10.
49. Mulleners WM, Chronicle EP. Anticonvulsants in migraine prophylaxis: a Cochrane review. Cephalalgia 2008;28(6):585–97.
50. Rasmussen BK, Jensen R, Olesen J. A population-based analysis of the criteria of the International Headache Society. Cephalalgia 1991;11:129–34.
51. Iversen HK, Langemark M, Andersson PG, et al. Clinical characteristics of migraine and tension-type headache in relation to new and old diagnostic criteria. Headache 1990;30:514–9.
52. Olesen J, Lipton RB. Headache classification update 2004. Curr Opin Neurol 2004;17(3):275–82.
53. Holte KA, Vasseljen O, Westgaard RH. Exploring perceived tension as a response to psychosocial work stress. Scand J Work Environ Health 2003;29(2):124–33.
54. Bertolotti G, Vidotto G, Sanavio E, et al. Psychological and emotional aspects and pain. Neurol Sci 2003;24(Suppl 2):S71–5.
55. Bailey DR. Tension headache and bruxism in the sleep disordered patient. Cranio 1990;8(2):174–82.
56. Ozge A, Ozge C, Kaleagasi H, et al. Headache in patients with chronic obstructive pulmonary disease: effects of chronic hypoxaemia. J Headache Pain 2006; 7(1):37–43.

Salivary Gland Disorders

Louis Mandel, DDS

KEYWORDS

• Salivary gland disease • Salivary disfunction • Diagnosis

SALIVARY GLAND DISEASE

Salivary gland abnormalities and salivary dysfunction are important orofacial disorders. Because of their anatomic location and subjective oral complaints, patients with such problems are usually seen in the dental office for evaluation and therapy. Inevitably, the dental practitioner will be required to make a diagnosis and institute care. Therefore, it is necessary for the dentist to be knowledgeable regarding the more common pathologic entities that involve the salivary apparatus, and also be familiar with the diagnostic and therapeutic tools that are available.

Since its establishment, the Salivary Gland Center (SGC) at Columbia University College of Dental Medicine has had the opportunity to examine more than 8000 patients with salivary gland disorders, ranging in age from infancy to the aged. Successful diagnosis has proved to be dependent on the organized integration of the information derived from the available diagnostic modalities: past history, clinical examination, salivary volume study, imaging, serology, and histopathologic examination. With the attainment of a complete work-up, an accurate diagnosis can be made and a meaningful therapeutic approach can be achieved.

Numerous salivary gland and/or secretory dysfunctions exist. This article highlights and defines the most common disorders seen in the SGC and indicates the current approaches to diagnosis. Improvement in diagnostic skills will avoid serious complications and lead to specific and effective therapy.

FALSE-POSITIVES

False-positive patients represent the largest group of individuals seen in the SGC. These patients feature a variety of subjective complaints and/or objective conditions mimicking a salivary problem. Because of their multiplicity, only the more commonly seen entities are discussed in this article.

Somatoform Disease

The SGC has observed that, despite their complaints, many of its patients do not have problems associated with their salivary glands and/or saliva. Instead, these patients have somatoform disease (SD), which can be defined as a psychological disorder

College of Dental Medicine, 630 West 168th Street, New York, NY 10032, USA
E-mail address: lm7@columbia.edu

Dent Clin N Am 55 (2011) 121–140
doi:10.1016/j.cden.2010.08.005
0011-8532/11/$ – see front matter © 2011 Elsevier Inc. All rights reserved.

manifesting as a subjective complaint with no organic basis. These patients have many bizarre and objectively nonsubstantiated concerns related to their saliva. Thick saliva, granular or gritty saliva, foamy saliva (a normal condition that results when accumulated saliva is aerated by tongue movement), slimy saliva, a need to constantly expectorate or swallow, and with the problem often limited to a specific area of the mouth, all frequently represent the impetus for consultation. Patients often state that they have too little or too much saliva, but this is not borne out by volume studies.

The history of these patients is a significant aspect in diagnosis. They frequently have histories of anxiety or depression and are being treated with psychotherapeutic drugs. Other common denominators include a burning mouth and altered taste sensation, often reported as metallic in nature. The psychotherapeutics, along with many other medications, are anticholinergic and cause hyposalivation when the glands are at rest. However, salivary stimulation produces normal volumes because stimulation overcomes the effect of the drug. Conversely, salivary volume in salivary gland disease is diminished in both at rest and in stimulated volume studies. This difference is the key to differentiating true hyposalivation from perceived hyposalivation. In determining salivary volume, the SGC uses the established criteria for measuring stimulated flow rates with a Carlsen-Crittenden collector (normal 0.4–1 mL/min per parotid gland).[1] The clinician should also be aware that some medications, as well as some systemic diseases, can alter taste.

There are other common factors shared by the patient with SD. Questioning may indicate that some oral event or dental procedure was the precipitating factor for the problem. Concurrently, many patients exhibit other abnormal oral conditions, such as bruxing/clenching or unusual facial pain patterns, that may have a psychogenic origin. Stressful work environments or problematic social relationships can be contributing factors.

With no demonstrable organic basis for the complaint, treatment requires reassurance and/or psychiatric consultation. Patients often resist this suggestion for help.

Masseteric Hypertrophy

Masseteric hypertrophy can be caused by constant bruxing, clenching, or continuous gum chewing. With enlargement of the masseteric muscle, the face develops a rectangular configuration (**Fig. 1**). Confusion occurs when these patients are misdiagnosed with parotid hypertrophy (PH). Clinical differentiation is possible because accentuation of facial ovality occurs with PH. In addition, when the palm of the hand is placed on the facial swelling and the patient clenches, the previously enlarged muscle becomes even larger and displaces the hand laterally. The condition is usually seen in young

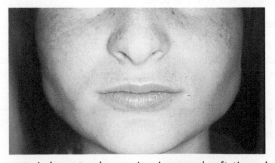

Fig. 1. Bilateral masseteric hypertrophy causing increased soft tissue bulk in mandibular angle areas.

individuals. Elderly patients with dental deterioration develop discomfort when activated masseters stress their dentition. Radiographically, bony hyperplasia, scalloping, and the development of an exostosis may be noted in the mandibular gonial angle region, and result from the stimulatory effect on bone from increased masseter tension at its insertion (**Fig. 2**).

For cosmetic reasons, botulinum toxin injections have been used to inactivate the muscle and cause muscle atrophy.[2] Muscle relaxants, behavioral modification, occlusal guards, and surgical muscle reduction are additional options for decreasing the masseter's bulk.

Lymphadenopathy

An understanding of the anatomic location of cervicofacial lymph nodes, plus a knowledge of the pathologic entities that cause lymphadenopathy, differentiate lymphadenopathy from sialadenopathy. Bacterial lymphadenitis, originating from a tooth or mucosal infection, is the most common cause of an enlarged lymph node in the SGC. Granulomatous and autoimmune diseases, metastatic malignancies, and lymphomas can also cause salivary gland area lymphadenopathies and complicate the diagnostic process.

The history, physical examination, and clinical findings, along with knowledge of lymphatic anatomy and drainage patterns, are mandatory for diagnosis. The sudden onset of a painful, circumscribed, movable nodule suggests a lymphadenitis. Neoplastic nodes tend to be persistent, painless, movable, but can be fixed when malignant, and enlarge over time. A simple method to differentiate a lymphadenitis from a sialadenitis is to observe expressed saliva from the suspected salivary gland. A cloudy saliva suggests the presence of pus from an infected gland (sialadenitis), whereas clear saliva implies an extraglandular process.

Imaging (computed tomography [CT] scan or magnetic resonance imaging [MRI]) is helpful to identify the presence of a lymphadenopathy. Biopsy, whether by fine-needle aspiration or tissue biopsy, affords the opportunity for definitive histopathologic study and diagnosis, and guides the therapeutic choice.

Neuromuscular Dysfunction

Drooling patients have an inability to manage their normal salivary volume, whereas patients with hypersalivation produce a true excessive salivary volume. The drooling problem originates from the neuromuscular dysfunction seen in patients with Parkinson disease, amyotrophic lateral sclerosis, demyelinating diseases, poliomyelitis, or

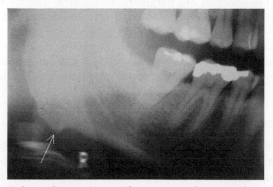

Fig. 2. Bony exostosis (*arrow*) in patient with masseteric hypertrophy.

a muscular dystrophy.[3] Patients who have received cervical radiation or who are developmentally disabled also drool.[4] Saliva accumulating in the anterior floor of the mouth, combined with a tendency for the head to lean forward, result in the propensity of these patients to drool.[5] Salivary volume studies testify that excessive saliva is not produced.

Relief can be attained with the use of antisialogogic medications (atropine, scopalamine, antihistamines), low-dosage radiation, botulinum toxin injections, salivary duct repositioning, and even surgical interruption of the nerve supply to the salivary glands.

Dental Conditions

Saliva has a protective effect in preventing dental disease. Patients with extensive dental caries are often referred to the SGC. An assumed deficiency in salivary volume or quality is the impetus for the referral. Patients with decreased saliva and caries related to Sjögren syndrome (SS) or who have received head/neck radiation are readily recognized. However, hyposalivation induced by medications does not seem to be severe enough to cause rampant caries. Patients with reflux disease regurgitate gastric acids and develop dental erosions.[6]

Once caries initiated by SS or radiation have been ruled out, suspicion should be directed toward an exogenous cause such as diet. Patients with an extremely high sucrose intake originating from soft drinks, sugared juices, candy, mints, or bubble gum have all been referred to the SGC. Despite the presence of extensive decay in these patients, salivary flow is normal. Their diagnosis is dependent on a thorough dietary history, which can suggest the cause of the rampant caries.

Treatment requires diet modification, good oral hygiene, fluoride therapy, and dental rehabilitation.

Paraglandular Opacities

Calcifications, when they occur in the region of a salivary gland, can be falsely interpreted as salivary stones. Differentiation is based on the absence of the pain and swelling associated with obstructive sialadenitis. Problems in diagnosis occur because asymptomatic stones exist.

Many lymph nodes are anatomically situated in close proximity to the salivary glands. Healing of such an inflamed node can result in calcification that mimics a salivary stone. Other causes of lymph node calcification include parasitic diseases, tuberculosis, sarcoid, metabolic diseases, and lymphoma. The key to diagnosis rests in anatomic knowledge and the absence of the signs and symptoms of sialadenitis.

A panoramic film can show spherical calcifications, varied in number and size, superimposed on the mandibular ramus (**Fig. 3**). A diagnosis of parotid stones is often made. However, the opacities are frequently tonsilloliths. The CT scan's axial view reveals these tonsilloliths to be medial to the ramus and associated with the pharyngeal space.

Other opacities noted in the area of the salivary glands must also be considered in differential diagnosis. They include aortic vessel calcifications, calcified thrombi (phleboliths) seen in cervicofacial vascular conditions, acne calcifications, and foreign bodies.

GASTROESOPHAGEAL REFLUX DISEASE

Interference with the function of the lower esophageal sphincter (LES), which normally guards against retrograde movement of gastric acids, is a major factor in the development of gastroesophageal reflux disease (GERD). In pregnancy, an increase in circulating hormones seems to decrease LES contractility, whereas anatomic changes

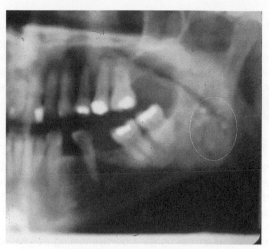

Fig. 3. Tonsilloliths (*circled*) superimposed on mandibular ramus.

associated with a hiatal hernia may physically impair LES function and/or clearance of acid from the esophagus.

With gastric acid intrusion into the esophagus, esophageal irritation follows and the subjective symptoms of heartburn develop (midline retrosternal burning sensations). Esophageal peristalsis may not be sufficient to rapidly clear the gastric acid and prevent esophageal damage. Limitation of the acid's effect seems to occur when the esophageal salivary reflex (ESR), mediated through vagal afferents, comes into play. Stimulation of the ESR causes episodic hypersalivation (water brash). With the inevitable swallow, the salivary hypersecretion lavages the esophageal wall and the buffering system neutralizes any residual gastric acid. Significant esophageal wall damage (Barrett esophagitis) from chronic exposure to the contents of gastric acid reflux is discouraged when the increased salivary flow flushes the esophageal wall and buffers the acid.

Many patients simultaneously develop episodic hypersalivation and heartburn. The precipitating factor (hypersalivation) for their visit to the SGC occurs when heartburn activates the ESR. A complaint of nocturnal drooling, causing maceration in the lip commissure area, can develop (**Fig. 4**). The supine sleeping position favors retrograde movement of stomach contents into the esophagus and saliva is stimulated. The regurgitation of

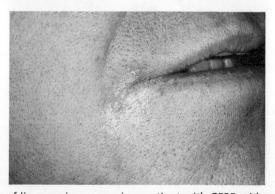

Fig. 4. Maceration of lip commissure area in a patient with GERD with nocturnal drooling.

gastric acids may extend beyond the esophagus and cause vocal cord damage and dental erosions.[7,8] During an episode of heartburn, salivary volume measurements substantiate the existence of increased salivation and serve as a diagnostic tool.[9]

Water brash can be ameliorated by treating the GERD, thus inhibiting ESR excitation. Prescribed medications for GERD include metoclopramide, cimetidine, and other antacids. Avoidance of spicy foods, alcohol, chocolate, and large meals, and elevation of the head during sleep have proved to be helpful in treating heartburn and the associated hypersalivation.

SIALOSIS (SIALADENOSIS)

Sialosis is characterized by a persistent, painless, bilateral parotid gland swelling with occasional involvement of the submandibular salivary gland. The parotid swellings are soft in tone, noninflammatory, non-neoplastic, usually symmetric, do not fluctuate in size, and often become a cosmetic issue. It occurs most commonly in alcoholism, but it can develop in diabetes, malnutrition, and even idiopathically.[10]

Autonomic neuropathy, manifesting as a demyelinating polyneuropathy, seems to be the common causal denominator uniting these disparate systemic conditions. The sympathetic innervation to individual secreting acinar cells is disturbed. This neuropathy results in excessive acinar protein synthesis and/or inhibition of its secretion.[11] Cellular enlargement then results from intracytoplasmic engorgement by zymogen granules and causes the clinically visible PH.[12]

Diagnosis is best attained by integrating the medical history and signs and symptoms obtained from the physical examination with data derived from varied investigative clinical modalities. Sialographic imaging shows a normal pattern of duct distribution and normal duct calibers. However, the ducts are distributed over an extremely large area, reflecting the clinically evident glandular hypertrophy. A CT scan of the parotid glands clearly shows glandular hypertrophy as the cause of the increased facial bulk (**Fig. 5**). In addition, the enlarged parenchymal cells replace the normally present lucent intraparotid fat and result in an increased gland density. Conversely, on occasion, a marked fatty infiltration of the parotid is seen. It is thought that, in the acute stage of sialosis, cellular hypertrophy is present, whereas the chronic stage is represented by a marked fatty infiltration.[13,14]

Fine-needle aspiration biopsy can be performed for histologic confirmation. Benign acinar cells can be seen. However, when measured, the individual enlarged acini

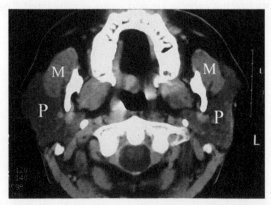

Fig. 5. Sialosis (alcoholism) CT scan shows bilateral parotid (P) enlargements overlapping onto masseter muscles (M).

reach diameters of 70 μm to 100 μm (normal 40 μm), further testifying to the cause of the clinical PH.

Treatment is directed at the underlying associated medical problem (alcoholism, diabetes, malnutrition). Therapy results in some diminution in parotid gland size, but the long-term prognosis varies.

BULIMIA NERVOSA

Eating disorders are a common problem. Bulimia nervosa (BN) is defined as induced vomiting after an episode of binge eating, and usually occurs in young women who have a self-image of obesity. As time passes, there is less tendency for the patient to limit the binge/vomiting cycles, and emesis is practiced whenever the patient becomes depressed, tense, or anxious. People with BN may vomit 2 to 20 times a day for a period of years. Because of the possible development of serious systemic complications from electrolyte depletion, diagnosis is mandatory.

Bilateral, occasionally unilateral, parotid gland hypertrophy is seen if BN episodes are frequent and persistent. The parotid's signs and symptoms are similar to those seen in sialosis. Bilateral, persistent, painless parotid swellings that are normal in tone and do not fluctuate in size are recognized. The patients become overly concerned with the cosmetic facial enlargement because of their distorted image of their body, and consultation is sought.

The pathophysiology causing the PH probably is identical to that seen in sialosis. Dysregulation of the sympathetic nerve supply to acinar cells results in intracellular zymogen granule, the precursor of amylase, accumulation, and a consequent enlargement of individual cells as shown by fine-needle aspiration and electron microscopy.[15] A use hypertrophy has also been suggested as an alternative hypothesis for the parotidomegaly.[16] Chronic autonomic stimulation of the salivary gland from frequent and repeated emetic episodes with hypersalivation is assumed to be the cause of the cellular enlargement.

A CT scan testifies to the presence of gland enlargement. Contrast enhancement and increased gland density from replacement of lucent intraglandular fat are also seen. The enhancement reflects augmented vascularity when emesis is actively practiced by the patient with BN.

Serum electrolyte studies are an important tool in diagnosing the secretive BN patient who practices multiple episodes of bulimia. Hypokalemia and depletion of serum chloride are often present and may require hospitalization, but are dependent on many factors including duration and frequency of emesis, use of adjunctive agents (laxatives, diuretics), and nutritional replacement.

Dental erosions, more severe than those seen in GERD, may be observed because the purged gastric contents and the contained gastric acid are projected against the palatal/lingual surfaces of the dentition. Another clue, a callused knuckle, may be present. It is caused by the incisal edges of the maxillary incisors as they rub against the fingers inserted in the mouth that are used to induce vomiting.

The need to stop purging is apparent. Usually, discontinuation of the vomiting results in normal electrolytes and a decrease in the size of the gland.[17] Most patients have difficulty following a treatment plan because of the underlying emotional problems. Therefore, psychiatric, group, family, and behavioral therapies should be considered.

ACUTE PAROTITIS

Acute parotitis (AP) is characterized by a sudden onset of pain and swelling in a previously normal parotid salivary gland. The primary cause of AP is dehydration in patients who are systemically ill and/or debilitated, immunocompromised, newborn, or after surgery in patients who have undergone abdominal surgery.

Severe dehydration brought about by inadequate fluid replacement and accentuated by sweating, blood loss, diarrhea, and vomiting initiates a decreased salivary flow. Salivary flow may be further decreased with the use of prescribed antisialogogic medications and the loss of mastication's stimulatory effect on saliva when the patient does not eat. These elements cause a significant hyposalivation with a consequent loss of the lavaging and antibacterial action of saliva. Poor oral hygiene also plays an important role.

With these components in place, an ascending ductal infection,[18] usually caused by *Staphylococcus aureus* originating from the oral cavity, can ensue and localize in the gland parenchyma. The swelling from AP is rapid in onset with unilateral, and occasional bilateral, parotid involvement, rarely affecting the submandibular glands. An indurated warm erythematous and painful parotid facial swelling develops. Intraorally, the parotid duct orifice tends to pout and a free flow of pus is visualized when the parotid gland is manually pressured (**Fig. 6**). Trismus, fever, leucocytosis, and toxicity are to be expected.

Clinical diagnosis is based on the presence of dehydration, hyposalivation, and the classic local and systemic symptoms associated with an acute suppurative process that, in this case, involves the parotid gland. Imaging (CT scan, MRI) of the culpable parotid usually shows a localized abscess and the increased cellular and vascular infiltrate associated with inflammation.

Treatment begins with prevention via improved control of fluid and electrolyte balance, and the prophylactic and therapeutic use of the more recently available and effective antibiotics. A conservative treatment approach is feasible because the parotid duct acts as an excellent drainage mechanism. Rehydration and systemic supportive measures are mandatory. If the patient does not respond to therapy, surgical incision and drainage are indicated.

CHRONIC PAROTITIS

Chronic parotitis (CP), the most common entity seen in the SGC, is readily recognized by its long-standing history of repeated transient episodes of unilateral and moderately painful parotid swellings. The intermittent meal-excited exacerbations, which may persist for hours or weeks, alternate with varying periods of asymptomatic

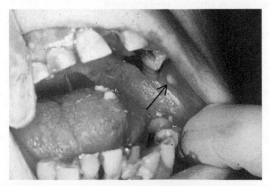

Fig. 6. Patient with AP. Intraoral view shows dry mucosa with suppuration present at the parotid duct orifice (*arrow*).

remission. With the continued waxing and waning of the parotid swelling, destruction increases and may necessitate gland extirpation.

Reduced salivary flow or blockage to its delivery may be the underlying cause of CP.[19,20] The resulting failure of sufficient ductal lavage facilitates an ascending duct infection from the oral cavity. Thereupon, bacteria damage the duct wall, with the inflammatory changes causing wall destruction and stricturing. The presence of these inflammatory strictures causes obstruction and salivary retention with duct dilations.

The bacterial activity that develops also results in the continuous development of mucopus plugs. Occasionally, a plug becomes lodged within the duct lumen and obstructs flow. The plug acts as a partial block, causing parotid swelling during meals when increased saliva is produced. Often these swellings rapidly subside when saliva seeps past the blockage or when the plug is flushed out by the salivary flow. Conversely, the swellings may persist for days or weeks and recede with minimal care only to return after varied periods of remission that can last from several weeks to several years.

During an acute episode, palpation reveals that the facial parotid swelling is tender and indurated. Intraorally, a flow of mixed saliva and pus can be noted exiting from the parotid duct orifice when the gland is aggressively massaged. With remission, a normal salivary flow is obtained. Continued recurrences from irreversible duct damage result in a downward spiral of symptoms with eventual marked involvement of the parotid parenchyma. Inevitably, the classic signs of an acute infection become manifest. Severe pain with eating, and swellings that do not recede between meals, associated with malaise and fever, are common complaints.

The history and physical examination are most helpful in diagnosis. However, imaging, particularly sialography, is indispensable to the diagnostic approach. With the intraductal injection of a sialographic dye, radiography clearly depicts the duct system. A sausagelike duct pattern indicates the areas of duct wall dilation and stricturing that result from the chronic infection initiated by an ascending bacterial infection (**Fig. 7**). Although the Stensen duct is primarily involved, the secondary ducts also show changes in direct proportion to the duration and severity of the CP.

In contrast with a sialogram's value in visualizing the duct system, the CT scan provides data concerning the parotid's parenchyma. Because of the inflammatory cellular infiltrate and fibrosis, the CT scan reveals that the parotid gland has become dense compared with its normal relatively lucent appearance.

A conservative approach can be used when caring for an acute episode and includes antibiotics, ductal irrigation, probing to break up blockages, and active manual gland massage, all followed by sialogogic agents to increase salivary flow

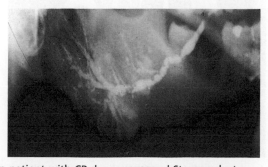

Fig. 7. Sialogram in patient with CP shows sausaged Stensen duct.

and impede further mucopus blockage. Retrograde duct injection of methyl violet, to cause inflammation with panductal fibrosis and gland atrophy, has been advocated.[21] A new approach using a sialendoscope for diagnosis, therapeutic irrigations, and stricture ballooning has met with success.[22] When the symptoms of CP are sufficiently severe, parotid lobectomy is indicated.

HUMAN IMMUNODEFICIENCY VIRUS PAROTID DISEASE (DIFFUSE INFILTRATIVE LYMPHOCYTOSIS SYNDROME)

Diffuse infiltrative lymphocytosis syndrome (DILS) is seen in a small subset of patients with human immunodeficiency virus (HIV). It is characterized by a CD8 lymphocytosis, bilateral parotid swelling, a diffuse visceral CD8 lymphocytic infiltration (usually the lung), and cervical lymphadenopathy.[23] The parotid swellings result from either a CD8 lymphoproliferative infiltration or, more commonly, from the development of lymphoepithelial cysts whose histopathogenesis is not clear.

Multiple cysts are usually found in each parotid gland (**Fig. 8**). They tend to be painless, soft, involve the superficial lobes of both parotid glands, and can cause gross cosmetic deformities. The cysts have little effect on HIV progression, although patients with HIV and DILS seem to have a benign disease progression compared with HIV patients who do not have DILS.

Diagnosis is achieved by ascertaining the presence of HIV via standard clinical and serologic studies. A diagnosis of DILS is made when the clinical finding of bilateral parotid swelling is combined with cervical lymphadenopathy, visceral lymphoproliferations, and, most importantly, the serologic demonstration of an increase of CD8 lymphocytes. The CT scan clearly shows the multiple bilateral parotid cysts or the significant lymphoproliferation associated with HIV-DILS.

In the past, parotid gland removal was the accepted treatment of choice. Because of the associated surgical morbidity, and because the consequences to the presence of these cysts were only cosmetic, no treatment became an option of choice. However, with the introduction of highly active antiretroviral therapy (HAART), successful resolution of these cysts has been accomplished. However, patients using HAART have experienced collateral damage in the form of a lipodystrophy syndrome. This syndrome is defined as a significant body fat redistribution, dyslipidemia, and insulin resistance. Fat depositions are often recognized, with the development of a buffalo hump and a thick neck. Patients can develop paraparotid fat depositions that clinically mimic parotid gland enlargement. A confident diagnosis is made when

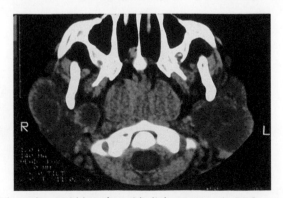

Fig. 8. Multiple bilateral parotid lymphoepithelial cysts seen in DILS.

the CT scan determines that the parotid area swellings are extraglandular and are caused by increased depositions of subcutaneous fat in the paraparotid region.[24]

SIALOLITHIASIS

Sialolithiasis, the formation of calcific concretions (stones) in the salivary duct of a major or minor salivary gland, is a common finding. These calcifications usually develop in the ductal system of the submandibular salivary gland, but can involve the parotid system and, infrequently, the duct of a minor salivary gland. They are found equally in both sexes, in any age category, and may be singular or multiple and even occur bilaterally.

Although the exact evolution of a sialolith is unknown, a nidus is required. The nidus is probably an inflammatory-derived glycoprotein gel. The gel creates a partial obstruction with salivary stasis, followed by a salt precipitation into the glycoprotein matrix.[1,25] Subjective symptoms eventually occur, testifying to the presence of an obstructive stone.

Classic symptomatology includes a history of episodic glandular swellings associated with meals, and present for variable time periods. The swellings may be painful, a suppurative flow at the duct orifice may be noted, and the floor of the mouth may be inflamed if the submandibular gland is involved. The suppuration is the end result of a bacterial infection, secondary to the stasis caused by the obstructing sialolith. Duct and parenchymal infection result and are manifested by glandular induration, severe pain, and systemic toxicity.

Diagnosis is facilitated when the clinical picture is combined with other investigative measures. Intraoral palpation, along the course of the Wharton duct or in the area of the Stensen orifice, may reveal the location of the stone. Standard occlusal radiographs visualize any stone in the anterior two-thirds of the Wharton duct, whereas an oblique occlusal view can be successful in showing sialoliths that are posteriorly situated in the region of the hilum. A periapical film placed intraorally over the parotid duct orifice reveals a parotid stone's presence in the anterior region of the parotid duct.

The CT scan is widely used for sialolith diagnosis because it is extremely sensitive to minute amounts of calcium salts that may be missed with a standard radiograph (**Fig. 9**). The scan can also establish the precise location of the stone and assess

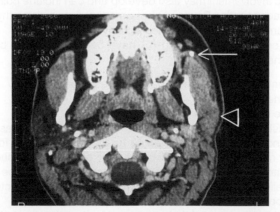

Fig. 9. CT scan shows small stone in anterior segment of left parotid duct (*arrow*). Note increased density, from inflammation, of left parotid gland (*arrowhead*).

the gland's status. Contrast should be avoided because a contrast-enhanced blood vessel can mimic the appearance of a stone.

Sialography also has a role in the imaging of a sialolith. Stones are seen as duct-filling defects with the obstruction confirmed by a proximal duct distension resulting from the salivary retention. The sialogram also depicts the extent of intraglandular duct damage and indicates the need for gland removal in association with the sialolithectomy.

Until recently, an intraoral surgical approach, to remove stones in the Wharton duct anterior to the mandibular second molar or in the anterior 2 cm of the Stensen duct, has been widely used. Alternatively, shock-wave lithotripsy can succeed in fragmenting stones into smaller pieces that can be spontaneously flushed out with normal or stimulated salivary flow. Failure can occur when some fragments are retained or when the sialolith is larger than 7 mm.[26] A laser beam technique, endoscopically guided, has also been used to shatter sialoliths.[27]

Although it has some limitations sialendoscopy, first described by Katz[28] and extensively described by Nahlieli and colleagues,[29] has diagnostic value and is the most popular means of noninvasive management of ductal stones. Optical and instrument miniaturization have made it possible. A flexible endoscope, diameter 1.2 mm, can be introduced into the duct. Advancement of the instrument is facilitated when the duct lumen is irrigated with saline introduced through the scope's irrigation port. With visualization of the sialolith by the endoscope, an attached Dormia basket is used to grasp and remove the stone. Recently, a combined lithotripsy and endoscopic procedure has been suggested.[30]

SJOGREN'S SYNDROME

SS is a systemic autoimmune disease that causes dry eyes and dry mouth, mainly in middle-aged women. Primary SS, or the sicca syndrome, is a solitary condition affecting only the lacrimal and salivary glands. Secondary SS is accompanied by other autoimmune diseases, usually rheumatoid arthritis but often lupus erythematosis or scleroderma. Although the pathogenesis is unknown, SS represents a complex activation of the immune system with B-lymphocyte dysregulation and hyperactivity playing a major role.[31–34] A florid lymphoproliferation into the exocrine lacrimal and salivary glands leads to parenchymal replacement and the clinical xerophthalmia and hyposalivation. Systemic involvement may also develop and can include pulmonary disease, vasculitis, lymphadenopathy, Raynaud phenomenon, autoimmune thyroiditis, gastrointestinal symptoms, and a peripheral neuropathy.

The following criteria for diagnosing SS have been established by an American-European consensus group[31]:

1. Patient awareness of eye dryness that may be accompanied by a sandy or gritty sensation in the eye
2. Dryness of the mouth and a history of swollen salivary glands
3. A Schirmer test to evaluate tear production attests to the decreased lacrimation
4. The labial gland biopsy, often referred to as the gold standard for SS diagnosis, shows one or more lymphocytic foci per 4 mm^2 of glandular tissue
5. Positive salivary gland involvement with hyposalivation can be determined by measuring salivary volumes with a Carlsen-Crittenden collector; in addition, a parotid sialogram usually shows a sialectic pattern (**Fig. 10**)
6. Serology provides evidence of the presence of autoantibodies to the SS antigens, SSA and/or SSB.

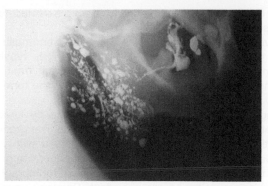

Fig. 10. Sialectic sialographic pattern (droplet/stippled) seen in Sjögren syndrome.

In patients with no associated systemic autoimmune disease, primary SS can be diagnosed if any 4 of these criteria are present, provided the histopathology or serology is included and is positive. A diagnosis can also be attained if 3 of the 4 objective criteria (Schirmer test, histopathology, salivary volume study, serology) are positive. Secondary SS is diagnosed when a systemic autoimmune disease exists in the presence of item 1 or 2 plus 2 conditions from the listed items 3, 4 or 5.

Prompt diagnosis and therapeutic intervention in SS are imperative because the local and systemic effects can be palliated. Continued observation is mandatory because of the propensity for the development of lymphoma. A primary oral concern is the inevitable onset of caries that results from the hyposalivation. Prevention of rampant caries can be achieved with the intensive use of fluorides. The use of pilocarpine or cevimeline has met with some success in increasing salivation. Salivary stimulation with sugar-free chewing gum and/or sugarless sour candy is helpful. Oral moisturizers and artificial salivas are available commercially.

Traditional systemic therapy includes hydroxychloroquine (Plaquenil), an antimalarial, which is widely used for treating SS arthralgias and fatigue,[32] and serves to increase salivary production.[33] Interferon α, cyclosporine, methotrexate, corticosteroids, and azothioprine have been used with limited success. Rituximab, an anti-CD20 monoclonal antibody, depletes B lymphocytes and seems to be the most promising treatment of the severe inflammatory manifestations of SS.[34] Nevertheless, despite the progress, management of SS remains a challenge.

SARCOIDOSIS

Sarcoidosis, a chronic multisystemic noncaseating granulomatous disease of unknown origin, has a special predilection for the lungs and hilar lymph nodes. It commonly affects young adults who present with respiratory symptoms and skin or ocular lesions. Patients with sarcoidosis have an increased tendency to develop lymphomas.

Salivary glands are susceptible to sarcoid. Involvement of the parotid gland, usually bilateral, occurs in approximately 6% of the diagnosed patients.[35] Submandibular salivary gland involvement is not as common, but 58% of the labial glands have been reported to show the pathognomonic granuloma.[36]

Salivary gland swellings tend to be firm, painless, and do not fluctuate with meals. A decreased salivation may be present. The salivary gland involvement may develop simultaneously with systemic sarcoidosis, or after the onset of systemic signs, or even as a herald before the development of systemic sarcoidosis.[37] Spontaneous regression of the swellings can occur.

Uveoparotid fever, or Heerfordt syndrome, represents an unusual clinical pattern of salivary gland involvement in systemic sarcoidosis. It is typified by a triad of symptoms that includes inflammation of the eye's uveal tract, bilateral parotid gland swelling, and cranial nerve involvement, usually in the form of a facial nerve paralysis.

A definitive diagnosis of sarcoidosis is best achieved by integrating the presence of noncaseating granulomas with the clinical data. The granulomas are characterized by tightly grouped epithelioid cells interspersed with a few giant cells, and with accumulations of lymphocytes at the periphery of the granuloma. Clinical data concerning the patient's medical history, chest radiographic findings, and results of the physical examination are important. Serology usually testifies to an increase of the angiotensin-converting enzyme. Gallium scintigraphy produces a distinctive pattern, the panda sign, because the radioisotope accumulates in the nasopharynx, parotid, and lacrimal glands and mimics the dark facial markings seen in the panda.

Observation is a viable therapeutic approach because spontaneous symptom regression does occur. Corticosteroids are the primary treatment of patients with decreased lung function or if the eyes, heart, kidneys, or spleen are severely involved. Infliximab, an immunosuppressant, has been used effectively to treat refractory sarcoidosis.[38]

PNEUMOPAROTID

Pneumoparotid is the forced retrograde inflation of air through the parotid duct orifice. The entity was first recognized when French Foreign Legionnaires created factitious cases of mumps by forcefully blowing into a small rigid container. The resulting increased intraoral pressure encouraged the movement of air into the parotid duct and gland. This refluxing of air through the parotid duct orifice is seen in wind instrument players, glass blowers, and persons who increase intraoral pressure by blowing up their cheeks consciously or as a neurotic habit or tic. Such habits have emotional overtones. It also is seen in cases of anesthesia mumps, in which it follows a troubled course of general anesthesia with excessive coughing and sneezing and the use of muscle relaxants. The increased oral air pressure from the coughing/sneezing, combined with muscle tone loss, facilitates the pneumoparotid.

The parotid swelling that develops can be unilateral or, less frequently, bilateral and can subside spontaneously. The sialadenopathy is accompanied by a sense of fullness or slight discomfort. Palpation produces the classic crackling sensation associated with a tissue emphysema. Viewing of the parotid duct orifice, as the gland is pressured extraorally, reveals a pathognomonic frothy and bubbly aerated saliva [39] (Fig. 11). This unique and key feature reflects the forced mixture of air with saliva contained within the limiting confines of the ductal system.

Chronic forced entry of air into the ductal system can lead to infection. The symptoms of a CP are then superimposed on the features of a pneumoparotid. A sialographic pattern of sausaging develops and reflects duct stricturing and dilatations. Autoinsufflation should be stopped to prevent these degenerative changes. However, this may be difficult to accomplish because the problem often represents an unconscious habit or occupational necessity. Treatment also involves both counseling and measures aimed at the problem of chronic infection.

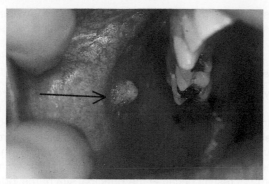

Fig. 11. Pneumoparotid. Aerated saliva exiting from parotid duct orifice (*arrow*).

RADIATION SIALADENITIS

Radiation to the salivary glands, significant enough to cause glandular damage, is delivered either by external beam radiation (EBR) or through the ingestion of radioactive iodine (^{131}I).

External Beam Radiation

EBR is widely used in the treatment of cancers of the oral cavity, salivary glands, lymph nodes, and metastatic lesions to the head and neck area. The therapy also includes surgery and chemotherapy when indicated. Of great concern to the dental clinician are the inevitable complications associated with irradiation. Salivary production by the serous acini is readily affected in 1 week with applications of 16 Gy.[40] The mucous acini of the submandibular salivary gland seem to be more resistant to irradiation and are only affected at higher dose levels. Some recovery of salivary secretion occurs if the irradiation is less than 26 Gy.[41] An irreversible loss of salivary gland secretion results from doses of more than 40 Gy, with residual glandular tissue functioning only at levels 5% to 15% of normal.[42] Doses of 60 Gy cause glandular atrophy and fibrosis with only minimal salivary production.[40] With such doses, osteonecrosis becomes a serious concern.

Hyposalivation is the inevitable result of EBR. The salivary consistency becomes viscous because the saliva's serous element is markedly reduced in proportion to the secretory production of the more resistant mucous acini. With loss of saliva's bacterial, protective, and buffering powers, mucositis, candidiasis, dysgeusia, dysphagia, and trismus can be encountered when cancericidal doses of radiation are used.

Diagnosis is simplified once the medical history is combined with the clinical examination. Treatment begins with the preventive measures that can be used when radiotherapy is instituted. Three-dimensional and intensity-modulated radiotherapeutic approaches are used to limit salivary gland radiation exposure. The cytoprotectant amifostine can also limit salivary gland injury.

Treatment of the oral conditions resulting from irradiation encompasses a variety of techniques. Aggressive fluoride management is required to control the extensive caries that develop. Pilocarpine or cevimeline, with the adjunctive use of sugarless sour candy or chewing gum, stimulate residual parenchymal tissue and increase salivation. Artificial salivas, moisturizers, and lubricant mouthwashes are available to ameliorate the discomfort that develops with a dry mouth. Antifungals are used if candidiasis is present. Oral hygiene has to be maintained and the patient must avoid dehydration.

Radioactive Iodine (^{131}I)

^{131}I targets the thyroid gland and has plays an effective role in the treatment of differentiated papillary and follicular thyroid cancers. Simultaneously, this radioisotope targets the salivary glands, where it is concentrated and secreted into the saliva. Dose- and time-related damage to the salivary parenchyma result from the ^{131}I irradiation. Salivary gland swelling and pain, most frequently involving the parotid glands, may develop immediately after the therapeutic dose of ^{131}I and/or months later.[43]

Direct injury from ^{131}I results because the principal site of the iodide transport into the saliva is the epithelium of the parotid's secondary and tertiary duct system. Parenchymal damage also occurs with the parotid's serous cells being more susceptible to the ionizing radiation than the mucous and serous-cell containing submandibular salivary gland. Almost immediately after ^{131}I therapy, transient salivary gland swellings and pain become a problem in 39% of patients.[44] This dose-related condition disappears with resolution of the acute posttherapeutic inflammatory process. Subsequently, many patients develop obstructive salivary symptomatology that is dose and time related.

The effect of ^{131}I on the excretory ducts and the parenchyma are independent of each other. The usual therapeutic ^{131}I dose varies between 50 mCi and 150 mCi. At these levels, duct wall damage causes salivary retention and gland swelling during periods of increased salivary demand. Often, these obstructive symptoms subside, remission occurs, but future recurrences can be expected. After 7 years, only 5% of patients have salivary gland symptoms.[44] Higher doses of ^{131}I are used when a more forceful approach is required to control an aggressive malignancy. Hyposalivation with its associated oral symptomatology usually becomes manifest with the higher ^{131}I dose levels.

Diagnosis of an ^{131}I-irradiated salivary gland is made by relating the medical history to the clinical findings. The extent of gland injury is best determined via a scintigraphic study. Abnormal variations in glandular uptake and/or secretory ability are observed.

Treatment starts with prevention and the use of sialogogic agents and/or cytoprotectants, such as amifostine, to limit ^{131}I damage. These preventive approaches have had questionable success. Therapy for the obstructive symptoms has included duct probing, increasing salivary lavage with sugarless candy or gum, and followed by forceful gland massage to flush the duct. Dexamethasone duct irrigations, to suppress the inflammatory blockage, are helpful. Oral dryness can be treated as previously indicated in patients who developed similar problems when exposed to EBR.

NEOPLASMS

In the United States, the incidence of salivary gland tumors is 1.5 cases per 100,000 people, with a mean age for a malignant tumor of between 55 and 65 years. Benign growths occur approximately 10 years earlier.[45] Most tumors involve the parotid gland (70%–85%), 8% to 15% develop in the submandibular salivary gland, approximately 1% occur in the sublingual gland, and 5% to 8% occur in the minor salivary glands.[46] Generally, the smaller the salivary gland, the more likely it is to harbor a malignant growth. From 15% to 25% of parotid tumors, 37% to 43% of submandibular tumors, and about 80% of sublingual and minor salivary gland neoplasms are malignant.[46]

Accurate clinical diagnosis of salivary gland tumors is dependent on a detailed history and clinical examination. Benign salivary gland tumors tend to be slow growing, localized, and painless. Palpation substantiates that they are painless, circumscribed, and movable. There is no cervical lymphadenopathy or facial motor deficits.

Malignant salivary tumors tend to grow rapidly and can be painful. They do not have well-defined borders, and fixation results when the malignant cells infiltrate into the surrounding tissues. Parotid malignancies often invade the facial nerve and cause facial motor loss. With sensory nerve involvement, facial numbness can also occur. Cervical lymphadenopathy testifies to the ability of the neoplasm to metastasize.

Imaging studies (CT scan, MRI, ultrasound) are key components in the diagnostic study (**Figs. 12** and **13**). However, an accurate preoperative diagnosis can only be obtained by examining tissue obtained from an incisional biopsy. A fine-needle aspiration biopsy can show cytologic data indicating whether the growth is benign or malignant, and may even identify the precise histologic tumor variety.

Histologically, the pleomorphic adenoma is the most common benign salivary gland tumor. Papillary cystadenoma lymphomatosum, or Warthin tumor, is the second most common benign parotid growth. The mucoepidermoid carcinoma is the most frequently occurring parotid malignancy; the adenoid cystic carcinoma is the most common malignancy that involves the submandibular salivary gland.

Surgery remains the treatment of choice for all salivary gland tumors. Benign parotid tumors are best removed via a superficial lobectomy. The benign submandibular gland tumor can readily be removed by excision of the gland, which is facilitated by its well-defined capsule.

Malignant lesions demand extensive surgery the success of which is defined by obtaining adequate margins around the growth. Cervical lymph node excision is performed because the nodes may have succumbed to metastatic seeding, or as a prophylactic measure.

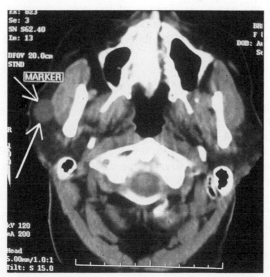

Fig. 12. CT scan illustrates presence of a well-defined benign pleomorphic adenoma (*arrows*) in the right parotid gland.

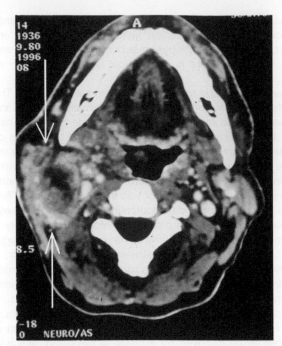

Fig. 13. CT scan with contrast highlights a malignant adenocarcinoma (*arrows*) with central necrosis (lucency) and surrounding inflammation in the right parotid gland.

SUMMARY

It is imperative for the dentist to be aware of the scope of salivary disease and simultaneously become familiar with the range of diagnostic modalities. Advances in diagnosis are constantly emerging, as exemplified by the recent introduction of the sialendoscope for the direct visualization of the major ducts of the parotid and submandibular salivary glands. The need to keep pace with such developments is obvious. Benefits will be realized in the form of early diagnosis and better treatment outcomes.

REFERENCES

1. Mandel ID. Sialochemistry in diseases and clinical situations affecting salivary glands. Crit Rev Clin Lab Sci 1980;12:321–66.
2. Mandel L, Tharakan M. Treatment of unilateral masseteric hypertrophy with botulinum toxin: case report. J Oral Maxillofac Surg 1999;57:1017–9.
3. Dray TG, Hillel AD, Miller RM. Dysphagia caused by neurologic deficits. Otolaryngol Clin North Am 1998;31:507–24.
4. Logemann JA, Bytell DE. Swallowing disorders in three types of head and neck surgical patients. Cancer 1979;44:1095–105.
5. Coates C, Bakheit AM. Dysphagia in Parkinson's disease. Eur Neurol 1997;38:49–52.
6. Dashan A, Patel H, Delancey J, et al. Gastroesophageal reflux disease and dental erosion in children. J Pediatr 2002;140:474–8.
7. Heidelbaugh JJ, Gill AS, Van Harrison R, et al. Atypical presentations of gastroesophageal reflux disease. Am Fam Physician 2008;78:483–8.

8. Holbrook WP, Furuholm J, Gudmundsson K, et al. Gastric reflux is a significant causative factor of tooth erosion. J Dent Res 2009;88:422–6.
9. Mandel L, Tamari K. Sialorrhea and gastroesophageal reflux. J Am Dent Assoc 1995;126:1537–41.
10. Mandel L, Vakkas J, Saqi A. Alcoholic (beer) sialosis. J Oral Maxillofac Surg 2005; 63:402–5.
11. Chilla R. Sialadenosis of the salivary glands of the head. Adv Otorhinolaryngol 1981;26:1–28.
12. Donath K. Wangenschwellung bei sialadenose. HNO 1979;27:113–8 [in German].
13. Rabinov K, Kell T, Gordon PH. CT of the salivary glands. Radiol Clin North Am 1984;22:145–59.
14. Mandel L, Patel S. Sialadenosis associated with diabetes mellitus: a case report. J Oral Maxillofac Surg 2002;60:696–8.
15. Donath K, Seifert G. Ultrastructural studies of the parotid gland in sialadenosis. Virchows Arch A Pathol Anat Histol 1975;365:119–35.
16. Ogren FP, Huerter JP, Pearson PH, et al. Transient salivary gland hypertrophy in bulimics. Laryngoscope 1987;97:951–3.
17. Vavrina J, Muller W, Gebbers JO. Enlargement of salivary glands in bulimia. J Laryngol Otol 1994;108:516–8.
18. Berndt AL, Buck R, Buxton RL. The pathogenesis of acute suppurative parotitis. Am J Med Sci 1931;82:639–43.
19. Bhatty MA, Piggot TA, Sommes JV, et al. Chronic non-specific parotid sialadenitis. Br J Plast Surg 1998;51:517–21.
20. Mandel L, Witek EL. Chronic parotitis diagnosis and treatment; case report. J Am Dent Assoc 2001;132:1707–11.
21. Wang S, Li J, Zhu X, et al. Gland atrophy following retrograde injection of methyl violet as a treatment in chronic obstructive parotitis. Oral Surg Oral Med Oral Pathol Oral Radiol Endod 1998;85:276–81.
22. Nahlieli O, Bar T, Schacham R, et al. Management of chronic recurrent parotitis: current therapy. J Oral Maxillofac Surg 2004;62:1150–5.
23. Itescu S, Brancato LJ, Buxbaum J, et al. A diffuse infiltrative CD8 lymphocytosis syndrome in human immunodeficiency virus (HIV) infection; a host immune response associated with HLA-DR5. Ann Intern Med 1990;112:3–10.
24. Mandel L, Alfi D. Drug-induced paraparotid fat deposition in patients with HIV. J Am Dent Assoc 2008;139:152–7.
25. Bodner L, Fliss DM. Parotid and submandibular calculi in children. Int J Pediatr Otorhinolaryngol 1995;31:35–42.
26. Capaccio P, Torretta S, Ottaviani F, et al. Modern management of obstructive salivary diseases. Acta Otorhinolaryngol Ital 2007;27:161–72.
27. Gundlach P, Scherer H, Hopf J, et al. Endoscopic-controlled laser lithotripsy of salivary calculi: In vitro studies and initial clinical use. HNO 1990;38: 247–50.
28. Katz P. Endoscopy of the salivary glands. Ann Radiol (Paris) 1991;34:110–3.
29. Nahliel O, Schacham R, Bar T, et al. Endoscopic mechanical retrieval of sialoliths. Oral Surg Oral Med Oral Pathol Oral Radiol Endod 2003;95:396–402.
30. Nahlieli O, Schacham R, Zaguri A. Combined external lithotripsy and endoscopic techniques for advanced sialolithiasis cases. J Oral Maxillofac Surg 2010;68: 347–53.
31. Vitali C, Bombardieri S, Jonsson R, et al. Classification criteria for Sjogren's syndrome; a revised version of the European criteria proposed by the American-European Consensus Group. Ann Rheum Dis 2002;61:554–8.

32. Kruszka P, O'Brian RJ. Diagnosis and management of Sjogren Syndrome. Am Fam Physician 2009;79:465–70, 72.
33. Rihl M, Ulbricht K, Schmidt RE, et al. Treatment of sicca symptoms with hydroxychloroquine in patients with Sjogren's syndrome. Rheumatology 2009;48: 796–9.
34. Quartuccio L, Fabris M, Salvin S, et al. Controversies on rituximab therapy in Sjogren syndrome-associated lymphoproliferation. Int J Rheumatol 2009;2009: 424935.
35. Greenberg C, Anderson R, Sharpstone P, et al. Enlargement of the parotid gland due to sarcoidosis. Br Med J 1964;2:861–2.
36. Nessan V, Jacoway J. Biopsy of minor salivary glands in the diagnosis of sarcoidosis. N Engl J Med 1979;301:922–4.
37. Mandel L, Kaynar A. Sialadenopathy: a clinical herald of sarcoidosis: report of two cases. J Oral Maxillofac Surg 1994;52:1208–10.
38. Mandel L, Wolinsky B, Chalom EC. Treatment of refractory sarcoidal parotid gland swelling in a previously reported unresponsive case. J Am Dent Assoc 2005;136:1282–5.
39. Mandel L, Kaynar A, Wazen J. Pneumoparotid: a case report. Oral Surg Oral Med Oral Pathol 1991;72:22–4.
40. Ship JA, Eisbruch A, D'Hondt E, et al. Parotid sparing study in head and neck cancer patients receiving bilateral radiation therapy: 1 year results. J Dent Res 1997;76:807–13.
41. Eisbruch A, Ten Haken RK, Kim HM, et al. Dose, volume, and function relationships in parotid salivary glands following conformal and intensity modulated irradiation of head and neck cancer. Int J Radiat Oncol Biol Phys 1999;45:577–87.
42. Grotz KA, Wustenberg P, Kohnen R, et al. Prophylaxis or radiogenic sialadenitis and mucositis by coumarin/troxerutine in patients with head and neck cancer—a prospective, randomized, placebo-controlled, double-blind study. Br J Oral Maxillofac Surg 2001;39:34–9.
43. Mandel SJ, Mandel L. Radioactive iodine and the salivary glands. Thyroid 2003; 13:265–71.
44. Grewal RK, Larson SM, Pentlow CE, et al. Salivary gland side effects commonly develop several weeks after initial radioactive iodine ablation. J Nucl Med 2009; 50:1605–10.
45. Ward MJ, Levine PA. Salivary gland tumors. In: Close LG, Larson DL, Shah JP, editors. Essentials of head and neck oncology. 1st edition. New York: Thieme; 1998. p. 73–81.
46. Spiro RH. Salivary neoplasms: overview of a 35-year experience with 2807 patients. Head Neck Surg 1986;8:177–84.

Imaging Technology in Implant Diagnosis

Christos Angelopoulos, DDS, MS[a],*, Tara Aghaloo, DDS, MD, PhD[b]

KEYWORDS

- Cone beam • Dental implant • Computed tomography
- Radiography

It is generally agreed that dental implantology based on osseointegration is among the most significant advances in dental science in the last 50 years. The success of implant surgery and restoration relies mostly on diagnostic imaging. This technology contributes to all stages of implant treatment, from presurgical site evaluation to postoperative assessment of integration, and long-term periodic evaluation of implant status.

Various imaging modalities have been used for dental implant assessment in the different stages of implant treatment. These include intraoral radiography (film-based and digital), panoramic radiography, computed tomography (CT), cone-beam computed tomography (CBCT), and others. Selection of the specific imaging technique should be based on its suitability for providing the diagnostic information required by the implant team (dentist, surgeon, radiologist) at different stages of treatment.[1] This article reviews the applications of different imaging technologies and their diagnostic contribution to presurgical evaluation, treatment planning, and postoperative assessment of dental implants.

Presurgical implant site assessment is a challenging task. Apart from clinical evaluation, diagnostic imaging offers the sole method of noninvasive analysis of possible implant locations. To fully evaluate an edentulous or dentate site for implant treatment, several objectives must be met. These include the assessment of normal anatomic structures at, and in the vicinity of, sites of interest; detection of pathology proximal to the proposed sites; estimation of the quantity and quality of bone; and determination of possible implant insertion paths as indicated by the angulation of the alveolar ridge.

The anatomic structures proximal to possible implant sites include the mental foramen, mandibular canal, maxillary sinus, incisive canal, nasal fossa, and existing teeth, all of which may limit the placement of implants. Specific pathology may eliminate the incorporation of certain implant locations in the treatment plan. Root tips, impacted teeth, or other pathologic conditions must be corrected before or during

[a] Oral & Maxillofacial Radiology, Columbia University, College of Dental Medicine, 630 West 168th Street, New York, NY 10032, USA
[b] Oral & Maxillofacial Surgery, UCLA School of Dentistry, 10833, Le Conte Avenue, CHS Box 951668, Los Angeles, CA 90095-1668, USA
* Corresponding author.
E-mail address: ca2291@columbia.edu

Dent Clin N Am 55 (2011) 141–158
doi:10.1016/j.cden.2010.08.001
0011-8532/11/$ – see front matter © 2011 Published by Elsevier Inc.

dental.theclinics.com

implant surgery. The decision to place an implant should be based on the knowledge that the selected site contains structurally sound bone that can support the integration process. The chances of successful implantation are increased by more bone being available for anchorage and distribution of masticatory forces. Cortical bone is best suited to provide support for implants. Accurate estimates of the alveolar bone height and width are mandatory for selecting the appropriate implant size and determining the degree of angulation of the edentulous alveolar ridge.[2] The assessment of the angulation of the alveolar ridge provides information regarding the proper insertion path of the fixture. The angulation of the alveolar bone represents the root trajectory in relation to the occlusal plane. Rarely does this bone angulation remain constant after loss of teeth.[3] The pattern of resorption of the edentulous ridge may give rise to undercuts and should be taken into account during treatment planning and implant surgery.

IMPLANT IMAGING TECHNIQUES
Periapical Radiography

Periapical radiography produces a high-resolution planar image of a limited region of the jaws.[4] Consequently, it may be used to evaluate the remaining teeth and residual maxillary or mandibular bone in the vertical and mesiodistal dimensions in a certain region of the oral cavity. Two intraoral projection techniques may be used for periapical radiography: the paralleling and bisecting-angle techniques. Although the goal of both techniques is to reduce image distortion, the paralleling technique is generally preferred, because the resultant image is less distorted.[5,6] The main principle of the paralleling technique is that the radiographic film is positioned parallel to the long axis of the teeth and the central ray of the x-ray beam is directed perpendicular to the teeth and film. This orientation minimizes geometric distortion and may be achieved using film-holding devices. Furthermore, keeping the x-ray source fairly distant from the teeth results in additional reduction in the geometric distortion and increases definition of the radiographic image.[7] The bisecting-angle technique is based on Cieszynski's rule of isometry, which states that 2 triangles are equal when they have one common side and 2 equal angles. In dental radiography, the central ray of the x-ray beam is directed at right angles to an imaginary plane bisecting the angle formed by the long axis of the teeth and the radiographic film. The 2 right-angled triangles formed are equal and consequently have their hypotenuse sides (long axis of the teeth and film) equal. Consequently, the radiographic image of the teeth has the same length as the actual teeth.

Periapical radiography is a useful higher yield modality for ruling out disease in the area of interest and is of value in the identification of anatomic structures proximal to the implant site. Periapical radiography may be helpful in determining the approximate height of the alveolar bone, the distance of the proposed implant sites from key anatomic structures, and the quality of the recipient alveolar bone by means of bone density and trabecular pattern.[4,8] Conversely, other authors[2,3] contend that bone density measurements should not be attempted from periapical radiographs and that significant concerns regarding the amount of available mineral in the bone warrant other methods. Also, Misch[3] considers periapical radiography to be of limited value in determining bone quantity because of the magnification. The imaging field with periapical radiography is restricted and its reproducibility is limited. Moreover, this modality is of no value in depicting the buccolingual width of the edentulous ridge. Periapical radiography is more often used for single-tooth implants in areas of abundant bone height and width. The use of periapical radiographs in the edentulous patients is limited.

Panoramic Radiography

The panoramic radiographic image is a curved slice of the maxilla and mandible of variable thickness, generated by a rotating x-ray source. This slice varies in thickness in the various panoramic machines and in the different areas of the oral cavity. Because of the specific image production principles, panoramic radiographs suffer from variable magnification, which is not the same in the vertical and horizontal planes. Equalization of the vertical and horizontal magnification is achieved only for a limited zone that lies within a curved plane called the central plain of the image layer or the focal trough. The focal trough is the zone in which structures demonstrate uniform magnification and appear more sharply on the radiograph. The focal trough shape and width vary from machine to machine. Structures that are positioned outside the image layer suffer distortion and magnification, the severity of which depend on the distance of the structures from the image layer. Panoramic radiography is a useful technique to evaluate the alveolar bone, the remaining teeth, and the location of neighboring anatomic structures (mandibular canal, maxillary sinus, nasal fossa) and to rule out the presence of other osseous pathology. It offers broader coverage of the maxillofacial region and allows comparison of contralateral structures. Panoramic radiographs are useful for the preliminary evaluation of the crestal bone height, bone quality and density, and cortical boundaries of the mandibular canal, maxillary sinus, and nasal fossa, provided that no positioning errors have occurred.[1] The panoramic radiograph is a 2-dimensional (2-D) image of 3-dimensional (3-D) structures. Consequently, it does not demonstrate the buccal-lingual dimension of the maxillofacial structures, and therefore, it is inadequate for estimation of bone width. Moreover, it is a flattened, spread-out image of curved structures, resulting in considerable distortion of the structures and their relationship in space.

Panoramic radiography has a variable magnification that ranges from 10% to 30%. Sometimes, this varies in different areas within the same panoramic image (**Fig. 1**). Also, image magnification is more variable when positioning errors are encountered. Misch[3] states that panoramic radiography is misleading for alveolar bone height, because of magnification and the spatial relationship of the anatomic structures proximal to the area of interest being of little use.

Panoramic radiography is, however, a fast, convenient, and readily available imaging modality, characteristics of which have made it popular with dental practitioners. Because of its popularity, clinicians have developed a means to compensate for recognized shortcomings and to correct for errors. Diagnostic splints incorporating metal markers with known dimensions enable the clinician to determine the magnification in the area of interest (see **Fig. 1**). Despite its popularity, panoramic radiography is inadequate as a sole means of surgical implant assessment because of the identified deficiencies. It may be used with other imaging modalities (ie, conventional tomography or CT) for a more adequate evaluation of the recipient site.[2,3,8]

CT

CT is a digital imaging technique that allows the operator to generate sections of the tissues of interest by using a finely collimated rotating x-ray beam and a series of mathematical algorithms. The resulting images are free of blurring and overlapping shadows of neighboring structures.

The CT scanner consists of a radiographic tube emitting a finely collimated beam directed to a series of scintillation detectors or ionizing chambers. The information

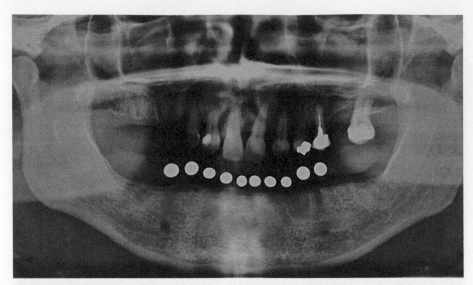

Fig. 1. Panoramic image for preimplant assessment of the edentulous mandible. A radiographic stent with opaque markers (metal spheres, 5 mm in diameter) was present in the patient's mouth during the radiographic examination. Note the different magnification of the various markers throughout the mandible.

collected by the detectors represents a composite of the absorption characteristics of all tissues and structures in the path of the x-rays.[4] This information is transferred to the CT machine in which the data of the multiple projections are transformed into an image. The CT image is displayed as a matrix of individual blocks called voxels (volume elements), whereas the square of the image that represents each block on the screen is called a pixel (picture element). Each voxel and consequently the pixel by which it is displayed are characterized by a numerical value that reflects its x-ray attenuation features, which is mainly affected by the density of the tissue and its thickness (dimensions of the voxel). This is called the CT number. The computer assigns a specific shade of gray or density value to each CT number using a matrix of gray shades, which comprise the image. The primary advantage of CT is complete elimination of shadows of structures lying deep or superficial to the structures of interest. Moreover, because of its high-contrast resolution, CT can distinguish between tissues that differ by less than 1% in physical density.[4] The density values of structures in the CT image are absolute and quantitative and can be used to differentiate tissues and characterize bone quality.[9] The axial images of the CT study can be resynthesized along different planes by including only the image blocks along a specific plane. The operator may select voxels of certain coordinates only, to generate new images. The stored data are realigned to create images based on the diagnostic needs of the operator. This is called multiplanar imaging and allows the structures of interest to be viewed in different planes, depending on the specific diagnostic needs. CT can provide images with a 3-D perspective by using information derived from axial images of the structures of interest. The computer realigns the voxels of the axial scans in such a way that voxels are relocated in space in a position relative to one another. To create a 3-D effect, only the voxels that represent the surface of an object scanned are projected onto the monitor. This provides a *solid* appearance to the structures of interest. Also, the surface pixels are illuminated on screen as if a light source was present in front of the viewer. Thus, pixels that are close to the light source appear brighter than those further away. The more posteriorly the voxels are located, the less they are illuminated.[1] This shading effect gives a 3-D appearance and depth to the scanned object, called surface rendering (**Fig. 2**). In addition to dental implant assessment, 3-D reconstruction has been used in cases involving treatment of pathology and trauma and in craniofacial reconstructive surgery for the treatment of congenital anomalies.

The development and widespread use of dental implants created the need for more specialized imaging protocols and multiplanar reformatting software programs that would consider the uniqueness of the maxillofacial region and the specific demands of implant surgery. Consequently, several proprietary programs that display multiple panoramic and cross-sectional images soon became available. Although the programs may differ from manufacturer to manufacturer, the following guidelines generally apply. After the acquisition of axial images, a curvilinear line is drawn on the representative axial image along the alveolar ridge (dentate and edentulous) in the midridge region. This line defines the plane and location of the panoramic reformatted images. The cross-sectional images are defined by multiple numbered lines that the software automatically places perpendicular to the curvilinear line (**Fig. 3**). The space between the cross-sectional images can be varied. If a radiographic splint with opaque markers representing the proposed implant sites is used during the scan, the areas of interest are easily identified.[10] Reformatted cross-sectional imaging with dental CT software results in images that meet almost all the requirements of presurgical implant site evaluation that were discussed earlier.

CBCT

The different imaging modalities discussed earlier provide answers to some of the diagnostic needs of implant therapy. Panoramic and intraoral radiography only provide 2-D information, not the 3-D information ideally required for implant planning. Also, their accuracy is strongly dependent on the skill and experience of the operator. CT has the potential to provide the required information with remarkable accuracy; however, it was only rarely used in dental medicine. Moreover, radiation exposure is

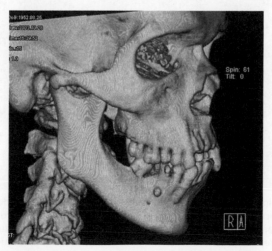

Fig. 2. 3-D reconstruction of the facial skeleton illustrating the surface only of the hard tissues, called surface rendering.

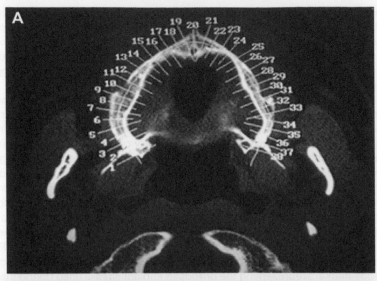

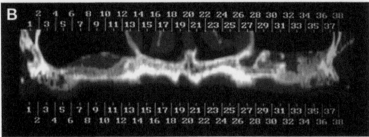

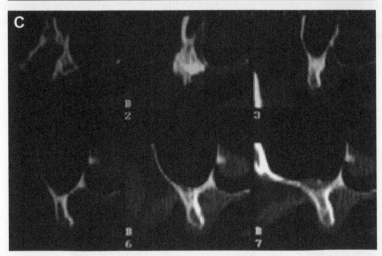

Fig. 3. (*A*) CT axial image demonstrating the curvilinear line along the edentulous maxillary ridge and perpendicular lines (numbered) indicating the reconstructed cross-sections. (*B*) Reconstructed panoramic slice along the curvilinear line depicted in (*A*). Numbers above and below the image represent the location of the reconstructed cross-sectional cuts and are correlated with the numbers in (*A*). (*C*) A sample of a few cross-sectional images selected from the series of images from the edentulous maxilla shown in (*A*) and (*B*).

fairly high, especially with older CT technology. The gap between traditional dental imaging modalities and CT was bridged with the introduction of CBCT.

CBCT uses a rotating x-ray source that generates a conically shaped beam, the width of which can be modified to fit variable-sized imaging volumes ranging from one-half of a dental arch to the entire head. The attenuated x-ray energy is acquired by a single detector with only one revolution around the patient's head (in most CBCT systems). Similarly to CT, the diagnostic information is collected by means of x-ray attenuation from the voxels of the imaging volume (numerous small cubes within the imaging volume discussed earlier). These data are collected by a single detector and converted to shades of gray as is seen in CT. The primary difference between CT and CBCT in terms of the acquisition process is that the imaging data are acquired from the entire volume at once (one revolution) in CBCT, instead of stacks of slices (multiple revolutions) as occurs in CT.

The introduction of CBCT in dentistry almost 10 years ago is closely linked to a new paradigm in maxillofacial diagnosis called interactive diagnostic imaging. This has its foundations in the concept of multiplanar imaging/reformatting that was established in medical imaging (discussed earlier). CBCT allows for the reconstruction of various images in any plane, flat or curved, by selectively realigning the imaging data (voxels). This property is linked directly to the fundamentals of CBCT data acquisition, which can be considered volumetric. In essence, the information stored in a CBCT scan can be used to generate and display reformatted images of different types using portions or all of the data. The standard display mode is *planar imaging* (sequences of slices in different planes, axial, coronal, and sagittal, throughout the volume). If the user desires a panoramic image from the volumetric data, this can be accomplished by carefully selecting (with a cursor) an uninterrupted sequence of voxels along a curved plane in the maxilla or mandible. The resulting image is a reflection of the voxels in the selected plane. If the user selects the surface-only voxels to be displayed, then a 3-D view is produced (surface and volume rendering). Although multiplanar imaging is not a new concept in medical imaging, in most cases, the reconstructed images were recorded on static media, such as film or paper, without any potential for interaction.[11] CBCT technology allowed interactive diagnosis, because the operator could now control the retrieval of diagnostic information. This has promoted interactive diagnosis, whereby the user can access much more information about each patient.

HOW DOES CBCT HELP?

Although CBCT has been used for preoperative and postoperative dental implant assessment, its contribution to the former is well documented in the literature. CBCT contributes to preimplant evaluation in various ways. The first and most important includes diagnostic considerations of the proposed implant site.

Preimplant Evaluation: Diagnostic Considerations

The clinician must know if an edentulous location is suitable for implant placement. Based on the concept of multiplanar reformatting described earlier, the proprietary software available with all CBCT scanners can provide multiple reconstructions, including sequential panoramic, cross-sectional, sagittal, and other type of images of the proposed implant sites or sites. For most scanners, these images are of variable thickness based on user preferences (**Figs. 4** and **5**). These images represent the interaction in the CBCT machine. These reconstructions are the result of proper selection and handling of voxels in order for special images to be generated. Once the reformatted images are available, a series of interactive applications are at the user's

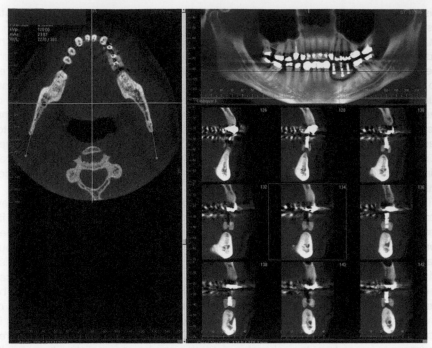

Fig. 4. Standard display format for the i-CAT CBCT scanner (Imaging Sciences International, Hatfield, PA, USA), including axial and panoramic reformatted images and a series of cross-sectional images, which can be scrolled throughout the maxilla/mandible.

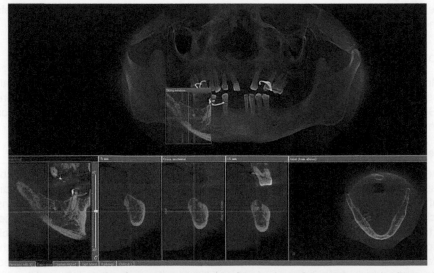

Fig. 5. Display format for the scanner GALILEOS (Sirona Dental Systems, Inc, Charlotte, NC, USA), which includes sagittal images in addition to cross-sectional images.

disposal, including measurement tools that provide alveolar bone height and width estimates (**Fig. 6**). Estimates of alveolar bone angulation are also available. This information assists in selecting the proper fixture as relating to osseous dimensions and insertion path. One important question is the accuracy of these measurements, because implant surgeons rely on them in different ways. A CBCT image is similar to a conventional projectional image, in that it casts a magnified shadow of the structures of interest because of the geometry of the x-ray beam. However, CBCT manufacturers incorporate advanced mathematical algorithms that are applied after image acquisition, so that when the data are projected on screen, the images are already corrected for magnification. These measurements have been found to be very accurate for most CBCT scanners currently on the market. In fact, the estimated error in various diagnostic tests involving accuracy of measurements with different CBCT scanners was reported to be between 5% to 12%.[12–14]

Dental implants are frequently placed in the jaws proximal to important anatomic structures that are to be preserved or respected during implant placement. The mandibular canals, mental foramina, fossae of the submandibular glands, lingual foramina, and neighboring teeth are some of these structures in the mandible. The nasal cavity, maxillary sinuses, nasopalatine canal, and neighboring teeth are some of the anatomic structures in the maxilla that may pose limitations to implant placement. Some of these structures are revealed with traditional dental images (panoramic, intraoral). However, the spatial complexity of some structures, (ie, the maxillary sinus, nasal cavity, and nasopalatine canal) limits the use of traditional dental images, even if they display the aforementioned structures. Anatomic complexity makes the use of sectional imaging a necessity.[15] Cross-sectional images identify undercuts and anatomic concavities in the alveolar bone. Existing undercuts may be accentuated after tooth loss, when bone resorption occurs. Depending on their size, these findings may limit or compromise a potential implant site (**Fig. 7**).

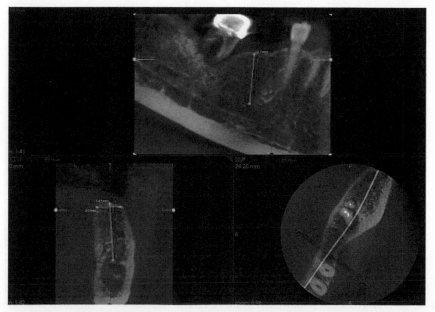

Fig. 6. KODAK 9000 3D (Carestream Health, Inc, Rochester, NY, USA): as compared with figures (4, 5), a different display. Measurement tools are illustrated.

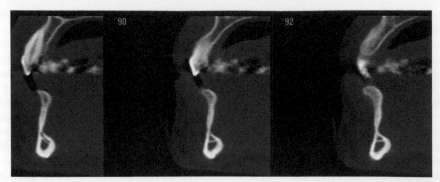

Fig. 7. Cross-sectional images in the anterior mandible as part of preimplant assessment. The marked lingual undercut has thinned the mandibular bone significantly. The anterior mandible is a region that usually demonstrates adequate dimensions for implant placement and exists even if the rest of the mandible suffered extensive atrophy.

Compared with traditional imaging, advanced imaging, including CBCT, depicts other anatomic structures, such as the mandibular canal, in greater detail. Moreover, the simultaneous display of multiple reconstructed images in different planes (axial, coronal, sagittal, and cross-sectional) increases the chances of locating the mandibular canal, even if it was not identifiable in some of the images.[16,17] To further assist the clinician in implant planning in the mandible, the path of the inferior alveolar nerve can be traced in the canal and evaluated in relation to the planned position of dental implants (**Fig. 8**).

The density and other characteristics of the alveolar bone can be evaluated with a CBCT scan. The thickness and integrity of the cortices of the alveolar bone, the

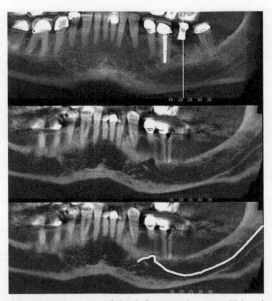

Fig. 8. Reconstructed panoramic views of the left posterior mandible: The mandibular canal may be highlighted in some of the software programs. Such a feature may be of great assistance during implant planning.

continuity of the alveolar crest and the integrity of the osseous boundaries with proximal anatomic structures, and the architecture of the alveolar bone are all considered determinants of bone quality. Bone density is directly proportional to load-bearing capacity, and implant failure has been linked to low bone-density.[18] Accurate estimation of alveolar bone density at the implant site would be of great benefit. However, density estimates provided by the various CBCT systems demonstrate much variation and inconsistency, even within the same system. This is mainly due to the high level of noise in the acquired images. Slight inconsistencies in the sensitivity of the CBCT detector in capturing the attenuated x-ray energies may also contribute to inaccuracies in bone density estimation. Also, the estimates are gray levels (brightness values) and are not true x-ray attenuation values called Hounsfield units (which are provided by medical CT scanners). Lately, several investigators have attempted to link gray-level values provided by CBCT to Hounsfield units.

Existence of pathologic conditions at the proposed implant site or in proximity to it may require identification and possible treatment, because they may have an effect on the outcome of implant surgery. These abnormalities include retained roots, inflammation in the maxillary sinuses, or other pathology.[19] The status of prior grafting procedures (sinus grafts, alveolar ridge grafts) can also be assessed by CBCT (**Fig. 9**).

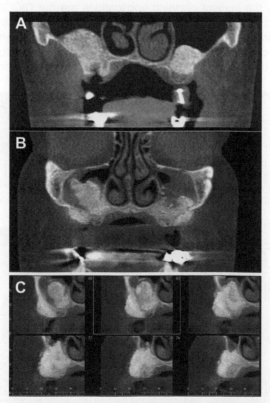

Fig. 9. (*A*). Homogenous, rounded bilateral sinus grafts demonstrating minimal or no inflammatory response. This appearance is consistent with a successful graft. Conversely, the grafts in (*B*), coronal images, and (*C*), cross-sectional images, are irregular in shape, undermined by inflammatory tissue, and fragments of the grafting material appear to float around the grafts. This appearance indicates failing sinus grafts, bilaterally. This finding may cause a delay in implant placement.

Preimplant Evaluation: Computer-Assisted Planning

CBCT data can be used for more advanced interactive applications, including planning for dental implants. A few manufacturers of CBCT scanners offer this service with proprietary software for each scanner. However, most computer-assisted planning applications are third-party and use original CBCT data exported to a universal format called DICOM (Digital Imaging and Communications in Medicine), which was introduced by the American College of Radiology-National Electrical Manufacturers Association. The development of this standard was in response to the growing need for standardization of the image format for export and transfer of medical images for CT, magnetic resonance imaging, and other devices. Compliance with the standard allows the various imaging devices to communicate with one another. CBCT data exported in DICOM format can be imported, viewed, and manipulated by various third-party applications. Some of these applications have markedly advanced implant planning, with the introduction of implant placement simulations, 3-D visualization, definition of the mandibular canal and other anatomic structures of interest, and advanced segmentation techniques (**Fig. 10**). In other software programs, the DICOM data of the CBCT scan are first converted to a proprietary format that is recognized by the application. This often requires a conversion that is external to the software itself. Because some of the implant planning applications are not DICOM-compliant, the DICOM data need to be converted into a format that is viewable by the proprietary planning application (ie, SIMPLANT, Materialise Dental NV, Leuven Belgium). Once the conversion is complete, a wide range of dental implant planning tools combined with realistic and undistorted views of the maxillofacial skeleton and the soft tissues

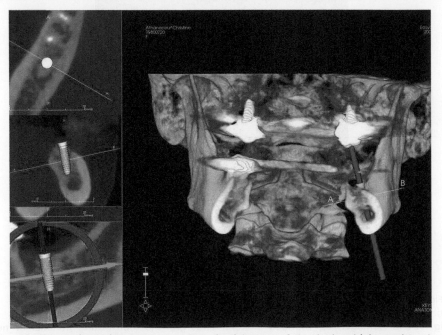

Fig. 10. The implant planning screen (interface) in one of the fairly widely used implant planning applications (InVivo; Anatomage, San Jose, CA, USA). Realistic implant images are maneuvered in space, so that the most appropriate insertion path is selected. The left side illustrates an axial, cross-sectional, and sagittal image of the proposed implant site. On the right is a 3-D image of the site of interest and the surrounding structures.

is available. These applications incorporate libraries of additional data, including manufacturer-specific computer-aided design-computer-aided manufacturing (CAD-CAM) files and libraries of realistic and proportional representations of dental implants as well as abutments and prosthetic appliances. These can be maneuvered and manipulated within the framework of the virtual world of 3-D imaging (**Fig. 11**).[20] Most of these software packages are continually updating their dental implant libraries in terms of implant size, type, available abutments, and other components, so that they can be useful for a variety of implant planning. In most cases, implant planning is visualized in at least 3 views: cross-sectional, axial, and sagittal. A fourth view of the dental implant in a solid or transparent 3-D virtual model of the maxilla or mandible can also be obtained. In this way, the dental implant is visualized in space, instead of only 2 dimensions. The goal is a high degree of precision in placement.

When several implants are planned, tools in the application can secure parallel orientation, and if the dental implant is to be placed at an angle, the angle can be determined so as to allow appropriate abutment selection.

Considerable information is revealed by removing the virtual bone, leaving 3-D representations of the existing natural teeth. This allows for implant placement in relationship to the teeth that are present in both jaws and can help prevent damage to natural teeth during implant placement.

Often, the clinician constructs a guide in which the proposed prosthesis (fixed or removable) is represented and the desired implant locations are identified. These

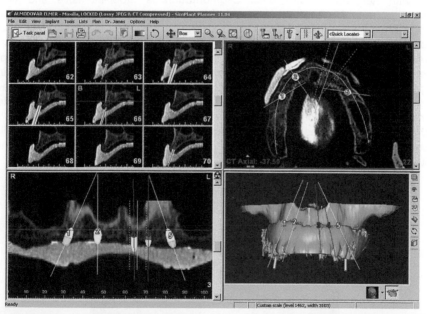

Fig. 11. The implant planning screen of one of the most popular implant planning applications (Simplant; Materialise). The 4 images show 5 implants placed in a simulated implant surgery in different views: cross-sectional (*upper left*), axial (*upper right*), panoramic (*lower left*), and 3 dimensions (*lower right*). In this case, a radiopaque radiographic guide was used to simulate the missing teeth and to guide proper implant placement based on the future restoration. Because the guide was of a different density than the rest of the tissues/structures represented in the scan, it could be segmented. This would provide the opportunity to have it removed or added based on need during planning.

radiographic guides include opaque teeth or other markers that have been placed in the desired position and orientation of the final restoration (**Fig. 12**). The virtual implant placement takes into account the shape, size, and spatial orientation of the prosthesis and allows for proper abutment selection.[21] All this occurs before the surgical procedure. The radiographic guide (3-D image of the guide) can also be virtually removed or added onto the 3-D image of the jaw. This allows visualization of the sites of interest, the dental implants, and the recommended prostheses to be visualized, together or isolated. In the same interface, the areas of interest may be viewed in different planes. To be able to isolate, extract, or add certain structures or objects to the 3-D model of the mandible/existing teeth/exceeding prosthesis, these need to be circumscribed and isolated from the CBCT data, most frequently by means of density or natural boundaries. This process is known as segmentation.

The anatomic complexity of the maxillofacial region makes visualization of important structures and their spatial relationship to others rather difficult. In such cases, diagnosis and planning may benefit from segmentation. With segmentation, data representing certain structures in an imaging volume may be isolated or removed from the volume, and this may simplify anatomic relationships and reveal diagnostic information that was obscured before removal. The segmented data can later be added back to the initial 3-D volume. In this way, the mandibular bone, if segmented, can be removed from its articulation with the temporal bone, to provide visualization of the glenoid fossa. Similarly, certain teeth, if segmented, can be removed from the jaw and illustrated with a different color or rendered transparent to assess the relationship with neighboring structures. Segmentation is labor-intensive and time-consuming, requiring an advanced level of knowledge of the application. The data from planned implant cases can be used for the construction of CAD-CAM surgical guides. The data are transferred electronically to proper laboratories to fabricate a CAD-CAM surgical guide (**Fig. 13**). This guide can be used during surgery to replicate the computer-planned procedure, avoiding anatomic structures and allowing for precise implant placement. Some of these proprietary software programs have advanced to the next step, in which provisional and final restorations are fabricated from the implant positions planned during presurgical workup.[22] Although this is only done in select cases, it demonstrates how new technology can markedly influence the surgical techniques in an effort to continue improving clinical accuracy while reducing complications.

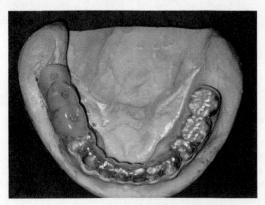

Fig. 12. Radiographic guide with opaque markers (gutta-percha) in the areas of interest. (*Courtesy of* Dr Reem Haj Ali, University of Missouri-Kansas City, School of Dentistry, Kansas City, MO.)

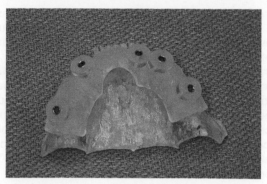

Fig. 13. A surgical guide applied on a maxillary biomodel. Both were manufactured by exportation of the planned case shown in **Fig. 11** with Simplant (Materialise). The metallic rings accommodate the implant drills during implant surgery and orient them into the exact location for the dental implants that were planned earlier during the simulated placement. These guides could be either soft tissue-supported or bone-supported.

The accuracy of dental implant planning may be further increased with currently experimental technologies, such as surface laser scanning data, which would be combined with the CBCT data. This would provide accurate information about the oral soft tissue (gingiva) in comparison to CBCT data alone, which provides only hard-tissue information. This may significantly increase the predictability of aesthetic implant-based restorations.

POSTOPERATIVE DENTAL IMPLANT ASSESSMENT

The factors that are primary determinants of implant surgery and the clinical outcome of implant-retained restorations are associated with the alveolar bone around the dental implant. The dental implant/bone interface (the contact of the dental implant to the bone) and the alveolar bone height in relation to the neck of the dental implant are crucial. A tight interface without the appearance of a thin radiolucent rim surrounding the implant and fairly distinct alveolar bone margins around the dental implant are signs of a successfully integrated implant (**Fig. 14**). However, bone loss around existing dental implants does occur, and literature has provided information regarding an acceptable rate of bone loss

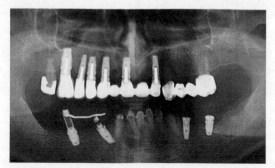

Fig. 14. Cropped panoramic radiograph, which was made for periodic evaluation of the maxillary dental implants. Note the tight interface between the maxillary dental implants and the alveolar bone that indicates a successful osseointegration.

over time,[23,24] In general, periapical radiographs made under standardized conditions can provide useful images of dental implants and the surrounding bone over time and can provide a fairly accurate assessment of the alveolar bone crest and possible marginal bone loss on the proximal aspect of the dental implant.[1] However, the marginal bone on the buccal and lingual/palatal surface of the dental implant, the proximity of the implants to the buccal and lingual/palatal plates, and the possible perforation of the plates cannot be assessed, because of the limitations of 2-D images. These limitations can theoretically be overcome using CBCT, which provides cross-sectional images in the region of the implant and, consequently, a more complete assessment of the dental implant. Unfortunately, certain artifacts (ie, metallic and beam hardening), that are inherent to CT, may obscure detailed evaluation of the dental implant/bone interface (metallic artifacts) or may result in ghostlike radiolucencies around the dental implants and other high-density structures that may imitate peri-implant pathology (beam hardening artifacts; **Fig. 15**). CBCT studies are often used in postoperative dental implant assessment when a complication is suspected.

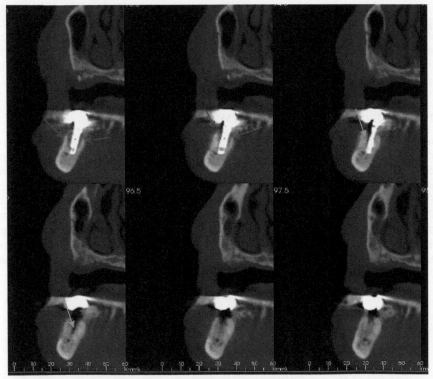

Fig. 15. Sequential cross-sectional images in the mandibular premolar region. The red arrows indicate a wide radiolucent zone on the buccal and lingual aspect of the implant, which is consistent with peri-implant inflammation. These osseous defects are not detected with periapical radiographs, because of their projectional nature. The green arrows indicate a linear radiolucent line in contact with the dental implant, which is suggestive of an artifact (beam hardening). This artifact is commonly seen around metallic restorations. The appearance is similar to peri-implant inflammation and must be interpreted carefully by the clinician.

SUMMARY

There is no doubt that implant-based treatment is one of the primary beneficiaries of advances in dental diagnostic imaging. Advanced dental diagnostic imaging, primarily CBCT, has contributed to far more accurate planning and has provided the potential for a significant reduction in complications.

CT technology has demonstrated a wide potential for predictable treatment results as far as implant placement and restorations are concerned and has potentially reduced operative time, morbidity, and postsurgical complications. Traditional dental imaging continues to play a vital role in routine postoperative dental implant evaluation, but the limitations of these techniques steer the clinician toward more advanced imaging methods.

Despite obvious progress, no specific selection criteria have been defined for preoperative implant site assessment and postoperative dental implant evaluation. Consequently, the proper image and image technology to be selected for the specific diagnostic task depends on the knowledge and experience of the clinician. Strict adherence to standards and guidelines, sound knowledge of the applications, limitations of this technology, and proper patient precautions are strongly recommended.

REFERENCES

1. White SC, Pharoah MJ. Oral radiology: principles and interpretation. 6th edition. St Louis (MO): Mosby; 2009. p. 597.
2. Reiskin AB. Implant imaging: status, controversies and new developments. Dent Clin North Am 1998;42(1):47–56.
3. Misch CE. Contemporary implant dentistry. 2nd edition. St Louis (MO): Mosby; 1999.
4. Goaz PW, White SC. Oral radiology: principles and interpretation. 3rd edition. St. Louis (MO): Mosby; 1994.
5. Bean LR. Comparison of bisecting angle and paralleling methods of intraoral radiology. J Dent Educ 1969;33(4):441–5.
6. Manson-Hing LR. On the evaluation of radiographic techniques. Oral Surg Oral Med Oral Pathol 1969;27(5):631–4.
7. Wuehrmann AH. The long cone technique. Pract Dent Monogr 1957;1–30.
8. Miles DA, Van Dis ML. Implant radiology. Dent Clin North Am 1993;37(4):645–68.
9. Brooks RA. Medical physics of CT and ultrasound: tissue imaging and characterization. In: Medical physics monograph no 6. New York: American Institute of Physics; 1980.
10. Som PM, Curtin HD. In: Head and neck imaging. 3rd edition. vol. 1. St Louis (MO): Mosby; 1996.
11. Scarfe WC, Farman AG, Sukovic P. Clinical applications of cone-beam computed tomography in dental practice. J Can Dent Assoc 2006;72(1):75–80.
12. Lascala CA, Panella J, Marques MM. Analysis of the accuracy of linear measurements obtained by cone beam computed tomography (CBCT-NewTom). Dentomaxillofac Radiol 2004;33(5):291–4.
13. Hashimoto K, Kawashima S, Araki M, et al. Comparison of image performance between cone-beam computed tomography for dental use and four-row multidetector helical CT. J Oral Sci 2006;48(1):27–34.
14. Hashimoto K, Kawashima S, Kameoka S, et al. Comparison of image validity between cone beam computed tomography for dental use and multidetector row helical computed tomography. Dentomaxillofac Radiol 2007;36(8):465–71.

15. Tyndall DA, Brooks SL. Selection criteria for dental implant site imaging: a position paper of the american academy of oral and maxillofacial radiology. Oral Surg Oral Med Oral Pathol Oral Radiol Endod 2000;89(5):630–7.

16. Stella JP, Tharanon W. A precise radiographic method to determine the location of the inferior alveolar canal in the posterior edentulous mandible: implications for dental implants. part 1: technique. Int J Oral Maxillofac Implants 1990;5(1):15–22.

17. Angelopoulos C, Thomas SL, Hechler S, et al. Comparison between digital panoramic radiography and cone-beam computed tomography for the identification of the mandibular canal as part of presurgical dental implant assessment. J Oral Maxillofac Surg 2008;66(10):2130–5.

18. Norton MR, Gamble C. Bone classification: an objective scale of bone density using the computerized tomography scan. Clin Oral Implants Res 2001;12(1): 79–84.

19. Hatcher DC, Dial C, Mayorga C. Cone beam CT for pre-surgical assessment of implant sites. J Calif Dent Assoc 2003;31(11):825–33.

20. Ganz SD. Computer-aided design/computer-aided manufacturing applications using CT and cone beam CT scanning technology. Dent Clin North Am 2008; 52(4):777–808, vii.

21. Ganz SD. Presurgical planning with CT-derived fabrication of surgical guides. J Oral Maxillofac Surg 2005;63(9 Suppl 2):59–71.

22. Bedrossian E. Laboratory and prosthetic considerations in computer-guided surgery and immediate loading. J Oral Maxillofac Surg 2007;65(Suppl 1):47–52.

23. Roos J, Sennerby L, Lekholm U, et al. A qualitative and quantitative method for evaluating implant success: a 5-year retrospective analysis of the Brånemark implant. Int J Oral Maxillofac Implants 1997;12(4):504–14.

24. Schwartz-Arad D, Herzberg R, Levin L. Evaluation of long-term implant success. J Periodontol 2005;76(10):1623–8.

Saliva as a Diagnostic Fluid

Daniel Malamud, PhD[a,b],*

KEYWORDS

- Point-of-care diagnostics • Saliva • Systematic disease
- Oral disease • Biomarker • Biofluid

Saliva is a clinically informative, biologic fluid (biofluid) that is useful for novel approaches to prognosis, laboratory or clinical diagnosis, and monitoring and management of patients with both oral and systemic diseases. Saliva is easily collected and stored and is ideal for early detection of disease, as it contains specific soluble biologic markers (biomarkers). Saliva contains multiple biomarkers, which make it useful for multiplexed assays that are being developed as point-of-care (POC) devices, rapid tests, or in more standardized formats for centralized clinical laboratory operations. Salivary diagnostics is a dynamic field that is being incorporated as part of disease diagnosis and clinical monitoring, and for making important clinical decisions for patient care.

Salivary diagnostics has been the subject of recent meetings and reviews,[1,2] and an overview of the principles of salivary gland secretion, methods of saliva collection, and discussion of general uses can be found in a report of a meeting published in the *Annals of the New York Academy of Sciences*.[3] These topics were updated in a subsequent meeting[4] and also in a recent textbook, *Salivary Diagnostics*, in 2008.[5]

Salivary diagnostics has evolved into a sophisticated science, and serves as a subset of the larger field of molecular diagnostics, now recognized as a central player in a wide variety of biomedical basic and clinical areas (**Fig. 1**). Molecular diagnostics feeds into a wide range of disciplines including drug development and personalized medicine (pharmacogenomics), and plays a major role in discovery of biomarkers for the diagnosis of oral and systemic diseases. This is especially true

This work acknowledges NIH grants DE14964 and U19 DE18385, the New York State Office of Science and Technology and Academic Research (NYSTAR), and the National Institute of Dental and Craniofacial Research and Drs Lillian Shum and Isaac Rodriguez-Chavez for their continued support and helpful suggestions.

[a] Department of Basic Sciences, New York University College of Dentistry, 345 East 24th Street, 916S, Schwartz Building, New York, NY 10010, USA
[b] Department of Infectious Diseases, New York University School of Medicine, New York, NY, USA
* Corresponding author. Department of Basic Sciences, New York University College of Dentistry, 345 East 24th Street, 916S, Schwartz Building, New York, NY 10010.
E-mail address: daniel.malamud@nyu.edu

Dent Clin N Am 55 (2011) 159–178
doi:10.1016/j.cden.2010.08.004
0011-8532/11/$ – see front matter © 2011 Elsevier Inc. All rights reserved.

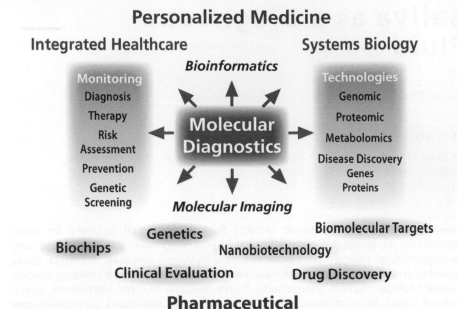

Personalized Medicine

Fig. 1. Overview of the centrality of molecular diagnostics to biomedical activities.

because most of the biomarkers present in blood and urine can also be detected in a sample of saliva. In this article the authors focus on the use of saliva and other oral samples for the diagnosis of systemic and oral diseases.

SALIVARY DIAGNOSTICS FOR SYSTEMIC DISEASES

Historically, systemic diseases are diagnosed via (1) patient-reported symptoms, (2) examination and a medical history obtained by a physician or other medical professional, and (3) chemical analysis of blood and/or urine samples. The patient's samples are typically sent to a remote, clinical diagnostic laboratory for determination of the levels of a broad series of markers including ions, antibodies, hormone levels, and a variety of disease-specific biomarkers. After some time (from minutes to days depending on the assay) the laboratory report is returned to the physician, and the results are then communicated to the patient. In general, oral samples are only taken if there is suspicion of an oral infection, for example a throat swab for *Streptococcus pyogenes* to diagnose "strep throat," or a mucosal biopsy for suspected oral cancer. However, there has been increasing interest in the use of saliva and other oral samples for the diagnosis of oral and systemic diseases. In a sense, the rationale is obvious. If it is possible to obtain similar or identical information with an oral sample that is easy to collect and that does not require invasive procedures, the need for a blood draw would become unnecessary; this is particularly important in several populations and situations, for example, handling pediatric and geriatric patients or when access to health care is limited in remote geographic areas where phlebotomists are unavailable. A recent survey reported that dentists believe that screening for medical conditions is important, and they are willing to participate when the sample is saliva as opposed to a finger-stick.[6]

Recently, the confirmation that an oral test for detection of antibodies to the human immunodeficiency virus (HIV) is as sensitive and specific as a blood test[7,8] has led to a large increase in HIV testing at a variety of locations including emergency rooms, sexually transmitted diseases clinics, community health centers, bath houses, and most recently in dental settings. The ability to accurately detect antibodies to HIV strongly suggests the potential to detect antibodies to many other pathogens. Indeed recent literature documents this for a large number of viral and bacterial pathogens.[1]

Oral samples that are useful for the diagnosis of systemic diseases include saliva, gingival crevicular fluid (GCF), oral swabs, dental plaque, and volatiles. Indeed, published data indicate the successful use of all of these types of oral samples to detect or predict susceptibility to systemic diseases.

The ability to accurately assess biomarkers in samples obtained from the oral cavity depends on the biochemical nature of the marker, the source and type of sample being taken, and the mechanism by which the marker enters the oral cavity. The most widely used type of oral sampling comprises a swab that collects a DNA sample. This method has been employed for many years in forensic studies[9,10] and more recently for single nucleotide polymorphism (SNP) analyses for mutations associated with specific diseases.[11] Although a DNA sample can be collected from a wide range of sites on or in the human body, oral sampling has been used most often because of the ease of the sampling procedure, that is, a buccal brushing that is placed in a stabilizing transport medium and sent off to a laboratory for evaluation. The commercial success of genotyping individuals for disease-related DNA sequences, while still somewhat controversial for its medical value, is not questioned for its scientific accuracy. Several companies have developed kits for collection of oral swabs for this purpose. Genomic profiles are returned within weeks that can predict ancestral origins and susceptibility to several diseases. **Fig. 2** presents examples of a selection of commercially available devices for collection of oral samples. Note that some of these devices (#3, #4, and #5) are shipped with a stabilizing solution for transport of oral samples to a testing laboratory. The salivette (#6) contains a cotton pad that is placed in the mouth and chewed; the pad is returned to its carrier and closed. The saliva sample is then recovered from the pad by centrifugation.

In terms of the number of publications, the second major use of oral samples is for the quantitation of steroid hormone levels. Assays are commercially available for cortisol, estriol, estrogen, and testosterone, and consistently provide accurate detection of these hormones.[12–17] However, salivary levels do not correlate well with serum levels in the case of conjugated steroid hormones. Thus, whereas dehydroepiandrosterone (DHEA) can be reliably monitored in saliva and the measurements reflect blood levels of the hormone, the sulfated derivative of the steroid, DHEAS, can be measured in saliva, but the levels are not correlated with serum levels. The reason for this discrepancy appears to be the route of entry of the hormone into the oral cavity. DHEA as a steroid can readily cross the phospholipid membrane of epithelial cells lining the blood vessels, so that elevated serum levels translate as elevated saliva levels by simple diffusion of the hormone. The addition of the charged sulfate group, however, impedes membrane transport and the substance detected in saliva likely represents leakage from the blood rather than diffusion. These observations raise the general issue of a qualitative versus quantitative assay for biomarkers. When qualitative (ie, yes/no) results are needed, as in the case of pregnancy or bacterial and viral infections, saliva sampling will generally be useful. When a quantitative result is needed, for example when analyzing glucose or DHEAS levels, one must determine the saliva/plasma ratio. If this ratio is close to 1, as it is for ethyl alcohol and unconjugated steroid hormones, then quantitative salivary testing is feasible; if not, then a quantitative salivary-based assay will not be suitable for that biomarker.

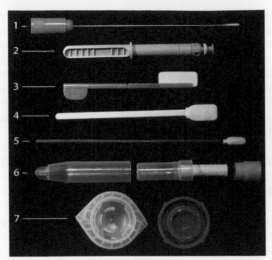

Fig. 2. Examples of commercial collectors for saliva. (1) BBL Culture swab collection and transport system from BD (Franklin Lakes, NJ, USA); (2) UpLink saliva collector from OraSure Technologies Inc (Bethlehem, PA, USA); (3) Intercept Oral Specimen Collection Device from OraSure Technologies Inc; (4) Aware Messenger Device for the Collection, Stabilization and Transport of Oral Fluid Specimens from Calypte Biomedical Corp (Portland, OR, USA); (5) Saliva Collection device for collection of DNA samples from children, from DNA Genotek (Kanata, ON, Canada); (6) Salivette from Sarstedt AG & Co (Nümbrecht, Germany); (7) Oragene saliva kit for collection of saliva samples for DNA analysis, from DNA Genotek.

The application of salivary diagnostics for systemic diseases received a major boost in 2002 as a result of a program initiated by the National Institute of Dental and Craniofacial Research (NIDCR), "Development and Validation Technologies for Saliva Based Diagnostics." This program was designed to establish collaborative research teams between engineers with skills in nanotechnology and microfluidic techniques and scientists from the oral biology community, to develop portable POC diagnostic platforms for rapid detection and analysis of oral biomarkers. Initially 7 research teams were funded by this program, and 4 of these projects were renewed in 2006. The currently funded teams are led by Dr David Walt (Tufts University, Medford, MA) who is monitoring chronic obstructive pulmonary disease (COPD) and cystic fibrosis, Dr John McDevitt (Rice University, Houston, TX) who is developing biomarkers for acute myocardial infarction, Dr David Wong (University of California, Los Angeles, CA) who is focusing on detection of oral cancer, and Dr Daniel Malamud (New York University, New York, NY) who is developing a multiplexed test for HIV, tuberculosis, and malaria. All of these projects use advanced techniques for rapid POC diagnostics for detection of the relevant biomarkers.[18–21]

A summary of selected molecules that have been accurately detected in saliva is presented in **Table 1**.

Salivary Biomarkers in Cardiovascular Disease

There are numerous published reports demonstrating that C-reactive protein (CRP) can be monitored in salivary samples; however, CRP remains a nonspecific inflammatory response factor that increases in many conditions including periodontal diseases.[51] Similarly, salivary immunoglobulin levels are known to increase in

Analyte	Examples	References
Hormones	Melatonin, insulin, epidermal growth factor, leptin	17,19
Steroids	Cortisol, androgens, (testosterone), estriol, estrogen, progesterone, aldosterone, DHEA	7,12–17,22–29
Antibodies	IgG, IgA, sIgA, IgM	7,22,29
Growth Factors	EGF, NGF, VEGF, IGF	30–34
Cytokines and Chemokines	IL-1β, IL-8, IL-6, MCP-1, CX3CL1, GRO-1α, troponin I, TNF-α	35–39
Nucleic Acids	Human DNA, microbial DNA, mRNA, siRNA, microRNA (miR-125a and miR-200a)	9,40–43
Proteins	100–1000 proteins	44–46
Drugs	Drugs of abuse (NIDA-5), ethanol, therapeutic drugs, anticonvulsants, antipyretics/analgesics, antineoplastic agents, antibacterial agents, bronchodilators, cotinine	47–50

Table 1
Analytes detected in saliva

Abbreviations: DHEA, dehydroepiandrosterone; EGF, epidermal growth factor; GRO, growth-related oncogene; Ig, immunoglobulin; IGF, insulin-like growth factor; IL, interleukin; MCP, monocyte chemotactic protein; NGF, nerve growth factor; NIDA-5, National Institute of Drug Abuse 5-drug test; TNF, tumor necrosis factor; VEGF, vascular endothelial growth factor.

association with coronary artery disease,[52] but once again immunoglobulins, particularly salivary IgA, are elevated in response to many local and systemic conditions. Recently, Floriano and colleagues[51] reported that a group of salivary biomarkers can complement findings of an electrocardiogram (ECG) following an acute myocardial infarction. These markers, including CRP, myoglobin, and myeloperoxidase, in combination with an ECG, showed a highly significant correlation with myocardial infarct patients as compared with healthy controls. Salivary biomarkers have also been incorporated into POC devices for the rapid assessment of cardiovascular disease (CVD) with potential association with distinct disease stages, demonstrating promising results in identifying CVD.[53] Elevated salivary lysozyme levels, a biomarker for oral infection and hyperglycemia, has also shown a significant association with hypertension, an early stage of CVD.[44] Despite the progress made in biomarker discovery, robust clinical studies are required to validate salivary biomarkers for CVD and its different clinical stages.

Salivary Biomarkers for Renal Disease

Walt and colleagues[21] and Arregger and colleagues[54] reported on a series of salivary markers that were associated with end-stage renal disease. The list of markers included cortisol, nitrite, uric acid, sodium, chloride, pH, amylase, and lactoferrin. In a subsequent study[35] by these same investigators, colorimetric test strips were used to monitor salivary nitrate and uric acid before and after hemodialysis. It was suggested that a salivary test could be used by patients to decide when dialysis is required, thereby eliminating unnecessary visits to a dialysis clinic.[55] Salivary phosphate has been successfully used as a clinical biomarker for hyperphosphatemia, which is an important contributor to cardiovascular calcification in chronic renal failure (CRF).[55–57] In this clinical study, 68 patients undergoing hemodialysis (HD) and 110 patients with various degrees of CRF were evaluated. Both HD and CRF patients had significantly higher salivary phosphate levels than healthy control subjects. Furthermore, evaluation of phosphate levels in saliva correlated positively with serum creatinine and the glomerular filtration rate. Thus, salivary phosphate may provide a better marker than serum phosphate for the initiation of treatment of hyperphosphatemia in CRF and HD. These results may also offer new approaches in hyperphosphatemia therapy by establishing measures to bind salivary phosphate in the oral cavity before saliva is swallowed.[56]

Salivary Biomarkers in Psychological Research

Stress and pain are often interrelated events. Investigators have attempted to distinguish them using a variety of model systems that induce either stress or pain, and subjects are monitored for changes in salivary biomarkers. Typical markers that have been identified include salivary amylase, cortisol, substance P, lysozyme, and secretory IgA. Pain responses in dental pulp have been specifically associated with neuropeptides including calcitonin gene-related peptide (CGRP), substance P, neurokinin A, and neurokinin P. Salivary testosterone levels have been associated with increased aggressive behavior and also with athletic activities.[58] Several reports relate cognitive behavior to levels of tryptophan and serotonin, the latter being monitored in saliva. It should be pointed out that for studies in psychological and behavior fields POC collection of saliva samples can play a key role, as a blood draw may induce both stress and pain in some individuals.

Salivary Markers for Non-oral Malignancies

The search for biomarkers for a variety of malignancies has been ongoing for decades. Once such biomarkers are detected in serum, it is a natural progression to look for these same markers in saliva. The ability to detect specific markers, particularly for malignancies that have few early symptoms such as ovarian and pancreatic cancer, would have tremendous impact on survival rates. Mutations of the tumor suppressor p53 were first reported for salivary gland adenomas in 1992[59] and were subsequently described in a pilot study of saliva from breast cancer subjects.[60] Subsequently, there were reports of elevated levels of the cancer antigen CA15-3 and the oncogene c-erB2 in women with breast cancer as compared with controls.[1,2,60,61] Chen and colleagues[62] identified the tumor marker CA125 in saliva of subjects with malignant ovarian tumors. Other studies have reported down-regulation of the tumor suppressor DMBT1 in mammary tumors in mice[63] and humans.[64] Zhang and colleagues[65] have identified 4 mRNA biomarkers that could distinguish pancreatic cancer subjects from pancreatitis and control subjects. It is likely that there will be an increased effort to substantiate and extend these findings in a variety of solid tumors in order to develop an early diagnostic profile.

Diabetes Biomarkers

Because of the large diabetic population, combined with the current epidemic of type 2 diabetes, an oral test to monitor blood glucose would be highly desirable. Unfortunately, while it is relatively easy to measure salivary glucose, because of the multiple sources of this material in the oral cavity salivary glucose levels do not correlate with blood glucose levels. However, several other approaches are under investigation. A recent report by Rao and colleagues[66] demonstrated a unique proteomic signature in saliva obtained from type-2 diabetics as compared with control saliva, with 65 proteins showing greater than a 2-fold change. Many of these proteins were associated with metabolic and immune regulatory pathways. While further studies are clearly needed, these findings suggest that there may indeed be a unique salivary biomarker profile associated with diabetes. Another interesting approach to detect type 1 diabetic hyperglycemia involves measuring exhaled methyl nitrate.[67] These investigators demonstrated a correlation between blood glucose levels and exhaled methyl nitrate, presumably because of interaction of superoxide dismutase with nitric oxide as a by-product of elevated oxidative reactions.

Finally, Strauss and colleagues[68] have proposed using gingival crevicular blood as a measure of blood glucose. In a study of 54 subjects, blood obtained during a routine periodontal examination was collected and compared with blood obtained with a finger-stick. The study showed good correlation between samples collected from these 2 sites.

Saliva Tests for Forensics

Salivary tests have been used for a wide variety of forensic studies. Samples can be obtained from drinking glasses, cigarette butts, envelopes, and other sources, then used to detect blood-group substances or salivary genetic proteins (primarily proline-rich protein polymorphisms). Approximately 85% of individuals secrete blood-group antigens in their saliva, including A, B, H, and Lewis antigens, that have been used for identification of individuals in both criminal cases and paternity law suits. With the widespread use of DNA testing, samples of DNA taken from the buccal surface with an oral swab can be easily obtained by untrained individuals without the need for a phlebotomist. Saliva is often present at crime scenes, along with other body fluids, and because DNA is relatively stable in the dry state, these samples can be used to place an individual at the scene of a crime.

Salivary Diagnostics for Autoimmune Diseases

Major rheumatoid factor diseases include lupus erythematosis, scleroderma, and Sjögren's syndrome. These autoimmune diseases are characterized by the production of autoantibodies that attack healthy tissue. Sjögren's syndrome is a disease characterized by dryness of the eyes and mouth,[69] and may occur as a primary or a secondary disease. The clinical symptoms in the primary form are more restricted and are associated with lacrimal and salivary gland dryness. In secondary Sjögren's syndrome, patients undergo one of the aforementioned autoimmune diseases before Sjögren symptoms develop. In contrast, primary Sjögren's syndrome (pSS) occurs by itself and is the third most common autoimmune disease, with a reported prevalence between 0.05% and 4.8%,[70] mostly (90%) occurring in women.

For decades, the pSS diagnosis has been based on oral examination, detection of blood biomarkers (autoantibodies to self-antigens [SS-A and SS-B]), rheumatoid factor, and antinuclear antibodies, and by obtaining a confirmatory salivary gland biopsy.[71,72] Patients with pSS have a 40-times higher risk of developing lymphoma, a fatal lymphocytic cancer. By contrast, patients with secondary Sjögren's syndrome tend to have more health problems because they suffer from a primary condition as well as Sjögren's syndrome. These patients are also less likely to have the antibodies associated with the pSS.

More recently, a panel of salivary biomarkers that can distinguish pSS patients from healthy subjects has been reported by Hu and colleagues.[73] Using cutting-edge proteomics and genomics technologies, investigators searched globally for markers in saliva from pSS patients and healthy controls, and found that whole saliva (ie, the combination of saliva in the mouth plus saliva from the individual salivary glands) contained a series of biomarkers that could detect pSS. In addition, the proteomic and genomic profile of these salivary markers reflected the damage to glandular cells, activated antiviral immune response, or programmed cell death known to be involved in pSS pathogenesis. The value of these candidate salivary biomarkers for pSS diagnosis has been confirmed by quantitative real-time polymerase chain reaction (qRT-PCR) and immunoblotting techniques by the same investigators. Similar to pSS, the progress made in cataloging oral biomarkers derived from the salivary proteome has provided a unique opportunity and a novel approach for the future use of salivary diagnostics in many other conditions.[45,74–76]

Salivary Biomarkers for Infectious Diseases

This topic was recently reviewed[1,3] and is only be briefly summarized here. The previous review[1] identified 23 viruses that could be identified in salivary samples by specific antibody reactivity, antigen detection, or nucleic acid via PCR. These viruses include a large range of herpes viruses, hepatitis viruses, HIV, human papillomavirus (HPV), influenza virus, and poliovirus. Fourteen bacterial pathogens were detected (by antibody, antigen, or nucleic acid), including *Escherichia coli*, *Mycobacterium tuberculosis*, *Helicobacter pylori*, *Treponema pallidum*, and a wide range of streptococcal species. Nonviral and nonbacterial infectious agents including *Candida albicans*, *Toxoplasma gondii*, and *Schistosoma mansoni* were detectable, typically by antibodies to these infectious agents. These pathogens are responsible for both systemic and oral diseases. Tests for these and for many other pathogens are currently under development by a large number of commercial and academic entities, so that it is likely that additional salivary-based tests for infectious diseases will continue to emerge. Some of the common pathogen- and nonpathogen-induced oral diseases and the role of saliva in their diagnosis are now described.

SALIVARY DIAGNOSTICS OF COMMON ORAL DISEASES

The physicochemical and biochemical properties of saliva along with its complex composition endows this fluid with multiple functions, including: antibacterial, antiviral, and antifungal properties; buffering capacity for plaque acids; digestive activity (amylase, protease, nuclease enzymes) needed for food mastication; mineralizing agents for protection and repair of hard tissues; lubricant and viscoelastic properties essential for the maintenance of oral health; and protective and repairing fluid for mucosal surfaces. Saliva is a hypotonic biofluid composed of 99.5% water and 0.5% ions (eg, potassium, calcium, chloride, sodium, and phosphates), and organic micro- and macromolecules (eg, amino acids, histatins, cystatins, defensins, statherins, lysozyme, proline-rich proteins, carbonic anhydrases, peroxidases, lactoferrin, mucins, secretory immunoglobulins, and lipids, among others). The origin of these salivary components is diverse and complex, and they are not reviewed here. Whole saliva can be easily collected with stimulating agents (using paraffin for mastication, or using citric acid or sour candy drops on the tongue) or without stimulation. The unstimulated whole saliva is often used in diagnostics, as stimulated whole saliva contains a diluted concentration of biomarkers that may be difficult to detect.

Another oral fluid of interest for clinical diagnostics is the GCF, which is an interstitial biofluid or inflammatory transudate that flows out via the gingival crevice and contains: cells (desquamated epithelial cells, neutrophils, lymphocytes and monocytes, and pathogens such as bacteria); electrolytes similar to plasma (eg, potassium and calcium); and organic components also similar to plasma (eg, albumin, globulins, complement s, protease inhibitors, lactate, urea, and multiple enzymes). The GCF has a protective role in the oral cavity by removing potentially harmful cells, molecules, and pathogens, and also has an antibacterial role by virtue of its pathogen-neutralizing antibodies.

Many of the salivary or GCF-derived molecules are used as diagnostic biomarkers for oral diseases including oral cancer, and conditions caused by fungi (*Candida* species), viruses (HPV, Epstein-Barr virus [EBV], cytomegalovirus [CMV]), and bacteria (multiple species involved in periodontal diseases and caries). In many instances, pathogen-induced oral diseases have been reported as opportunistic or secondary infections, and are referred to as early manifestations of the acquired immunodeficiency syndrome (AIDS) in HIV-infected subjects. The frequency of many AIDS-related oral manifestations varies, but increases in the absence of highly active antiretroviral therapy (HAART), and may indicate inadequate HAART treatment, development of drug resistance, or therapeutic failure.

Salivary Diagnostics in Oral Squamous Cell Carcinoma

Oral squamous cell carcinoma (OSCC) is the most common malignancy of the oral cavity among oral cancers (eg, adenocarcinomas, lymphomas, sarcomas, verrucous or mucoepidermoid carcinomas, malignant melanoma, and Kaposi sarcoma), accounting for more than 90% of clinical cases and ranking among the top 10 types of cancers worldwide.[77] However, oral cancers have also been reported with less frequency in the oral mucosa, tongue, pharynx, lips, gums, palate, salivary glands, tonsils, and sinuses. Epidemiologic data have shown an increased incidence and mortality of oral cavity cancers in many countries.[78] The latter is associated with risk factors including tobacco, alcohol, oral pathogen infections, environmental factors, and poor oral hygiene.[52] Classically, clinical diagnosis of oral cancer has been based on visual and palpation assessment, followed by biopsy and histopathological evaluation. However, this clinical assessment has been broadened by use of magnetic resonance imaging and computed tomography[79]; toluidine blue staining,[80] and light-based detection techniques.[81] More recently, detection of biomarkers in saliva has emerged as a novel approach for the diagnosis of OSCC and its developmental stages including initial process, invasion, recurrence, and treatment. A comprehensive description of these oral cancer biomarkers has been previously described, including oncogenes (eg, C-myc, c-Fos, C-Jun), anti-oncogenes (eg, p53, p16), cytokines (eg, transforming growth factor $\beta1$, interleukin [IL]-8, IL-1β), growth factors (eg, vascular endothelial growth factor, epidermal growth factor, insulin-like growth factor), extracellular matrix-degrading proteinases (MMP1, MMP2, MMP9), hypoxia markers (HIF-α, CA-9), epithelial-mesenchymal transition markers (eg, E-cadherin, N-cadherin, β-catenin), epithelial tumor factors (CYFRA 21-1), cytokeratins (CK13, CK14, CK16), micro RNA molecules, and hypermethylation of cancer-related genes (p16 and DAP-K).[43,82–88] These biomarkers have been defined using molecular, transcriptomic, genomic, proteomic, metabolomic, and phenotypic techniques. However, further development and validation of these biomarkers is needed for routine implementation in clinical diagnostics to assist with early cancer detection, risk assessment, and response to therapies. Refinement of a panel of soluble salivary biomarkers will depend on their stability and accuracy of detection, incorporation into sensitive and reproducible assays easy to perform, high sensitivity and specificity to indicate specific diseases and their stages of development, easy quantification in the clinical laboratory, and cost-effectiveness integration into clinical diagnostic algorithms.

Salivary Diagnostics in Oral Fungal Diseases

The oral cavity of immunocompetent individuals contains resident microbiome coexisting under a delicate immunophysiological balance and including an important fungal component known as the oral mycobiome. The latter includes culturable and nonculturable fungi, some of which may be pathogenic, causing common oral diseases such as oropharyngeal candidiasis (OPC), frequently observed in immuno-compromised individuals. A recent study characterized the oral mycobiome of 20 healthy individuals showing that *Candida* species were the most frequently isolated fungi (present in 75% of participants), followed by *Cladosporium* (65%), *Aureobasidium*, *Saccharomycetales* (50% for both), *Aspergillus* (35%), *Fusarium* (30%), and *Cryptococcus* (20%).[89] There are numerous factors that can disturb the balance of microorganisms in the oral microbiome and mycobiome, predisposing individuals to fungal diseases, including: physiologic changes that occur in the geriatric and pediatric populations and during pregnancy; disturbances of soft and hard tissues caused by lesions or poor oral hygiene; prolonged use of antibiotics with a broad antimicrobial spectrum; extended use of steroids that impair the immune system; nutritional deficiencies in micro- or macronutrients; endocrinological malfunction associated with diseases such as hypothyroidism; chemotherapy- and radiotherapy-induced immunosuppression due to cancer; immunodeficiencies caused by pathogens such as the HIV or congenital defects such as thymic aplasia; Xerostomia; autoimmune diseases (Sjögren syndrome); use of prosthodontic appliances; and diabetes. Mycotic infections of the oral cavity show different etiology, pathogenesis, and clinical forms. Primary OPC has been described as pseudomembranous, erythematous, and hyperplastic; while secondary OPC has been described as a chronic mucocutaneous presentation.[90] OPC, being one of the most common oral diseases, occurs as a mixed yeast-bacterial biofilm infection and it is most commonly caused by *Candida albicans*. However, other *Candida* species are also seen in medically compromised patients with a history of liberal use of azoles.[91] Classically the diagnosis of oral mycoses, including OPC, is based on an oral clinical examination along with the collection of oral specimens (swab, sputum, or saliva) for clinical laboratory analysis. The latter involves in vitro culture to isolate and identify the etiologic agent, direct microscopic analysis for pathogen visualization, and histopathological staining to confirm the etiologic agent and assess the severity of tissue damage.[92,93] To date, saliva samples for clinical diagnosis of fungal infections are only used for pathogen isolation and not for direct clinical assay applications. The performance of a commercial enzyme-linked immunosorbent assay (ELISA) kit to detect *Candida*'s mannan antigen in oral rinse solutions has been reported, but further assay optimization is needed for oral specimens.[94] Experimental attempts have also been made to detect salivary IgA or IgG antibodies to *Candida*,[95–97] but immunodiagnosis remains elusive because of differences observed in sensitivity and specificity of different assays when detecting various *Candida* antigen preparations.

Salivary Diagnostics in Oral Diseases Caused by Viruses

Oral diseases caused by viruses are prevalent, including papillomaviruses (HPV associated with oral cancer—OSSC—and oral warts) and herpesviruses (EBV causing hairy leukoplakia and also associated with various types of lymphoid and epithelial malignancies; cytomegalovirus [CMV] causing opportunistic infections after solid organ transplantation, retinitis, gastrointestinal and neurologic disorders, and oral ulcerations; herpes simplex viruses 1 and 2 [HSV-1 and HSV-2] and varicella zoster virus [VZV], also causing oral ulcerations of the aphthous type; and human herpesvirus 8 [HHV-8] causing oral and systemic Kaposi sarcoma). These oral diseases have been more frequently reported in immunocompromised patients because of impairment of the immune system, especially those with HIV/AIDS not receiving HAART, which represents more than 70% of people residing in countries where the AIDS epidemic is most devastating.[98–106] On initiation of HAART, HIV/AIDS patients show lower prevalence of some of these oral diseases (hairy leukoplakia and Kaposi sarcoma), but other conditions continue or may be even more prevalent under HAART (oral warts, oral cancers, salivary gland disease, and oral lesions associated with immune reconstitution inflammatory syndrome [IRIS]).[107,108] The clinical diagnosis of the oral diseases and viral agents described here is based on clinical examination supported by confirmatory clinical laboratory testing, including histopathological staining of tissue specimens, microscopic visualization of lesions and pathogens, virus isolation from clinical specimens, and nucleic- and immunoassays for detection of viral and host biomarkers. For instance, the standard approach for HIV clinical laboratory diagnosis has been testing serum or plasma samples in a sensitive ELISA followed by a Western blot if the ELISA is positive. However, oral fluids have also been successfully used in laboratory diagnostics to detect HIV antigen and antibodies in different nucleic- and immunoassay formats such as qRT-PCR, ELISA, rapid test, POC, and microfluidic diagnostic devices.[18,109–116] In addition, HIV-neutralizing innate immune factors such as defensins have also been successfully detected in saliva using sophisticated experimental methodologies such as liquid chromatography-tandem mass spectrometry, which involves limited sample manipulation and can be easily automated.[117]

Experimental detection of HPV in saliva samples has utilized nucleic acid assays such as HPV DNA amplification by PCR,[118,119] and this methodology has also been used to detect different HPV types.[99] Antibodies to HPV have been simultaneously tested in serum, saliva, and oral mucosal transudate specimens, yielding promising results when using oral fluids, but further optimization has also been recommended as a reliable alternative to serum HPV testing.[120]

The EBV DNA load in blood and saliva detected by PCR has shown similar results in cohorts of HIV-infected patients.[121–123] The nested PCR technique has been used to consistently detect CMV in subgingival plaque, unstimulated saliva, and peripheral blood of patients with chronic periodontitis,[124] and it has been reported that saliva is as reliable as urine for CMV detection in large screening programs.[125] More recently, saliva specimens have been successfully used for direct genotyping of CMV strains in a new PCR-restriction fragment length polymorphism (RFLP) method, coupled with capillary electrophoresis fragment detection for genotyping.[126] Comparative nested PCR analyses of saliva and peripheral blood specimens have consistently demonstrated HSV-1 detection with similar frequencies in both types of samples.[101] Similarly, reliable detection and quantification of nucleic acids for HSV-1, HSV-2, and VZV in oral fluids have been reported. There is a new standardized liquid phase–based saliva collection system, followed by a fully automated viral nucleic acid extraction and RT-PCR, using commercially available in vitro diagnostics/Conformité Européene labeled molecular assays.[127] Lastly, shedding of HHV-8 in saliva has also been demonstrated using PCR and immunohistochemistry,[128,129] and HHV-8 load in blood, serum, and saliva have shown comparable titers by qRT-PCR.[130]

The simultaneous detection of viruses in oral fluids using different assays with multiple applications is an emerging field. Many of these assays are changing to incorporate multiplexing capabilities and to take advantage of nanotechnology approaches, yielding automated, reliable, and sensitive diagnostic devices. However, these novel detection systems require further optimization and validation prior to implementation in routine clinical diagnostics.

Salivary Diagnostics in Oral Diseases Caused by Bacteria

Caries and periodontitis are the most commonly known polymicrobial-driven diseases of the oral cavity. Periodontal disease is a chronic inflammatory process of the periodontium in response to bacterial plaque deposited on the adjacent teeth. Bacterial species form biofilms, destroy the alveolar bone and periodontal ligament, induce gingivitis, cause apical migration of the epithelial attachment resulting in the formation of periodontal pockets, and induce irreversible loss and exfoliation of the teeth. If left untreated, gingivitis may progress to periodontitis, leading to tooth loss and severe lesions of soft and hard tissues. Periodontitis is also linked to systemic illness, such as CVD and diabetes. Caries is also caused by bacterial plaque that in combination with fermentable carbohydrates produces acids (eg, lactic acid) that lower the pH at the surface of the tooth, compromising the enamel, dentin, and cementum, and ultimately affect the structural integrity of the tooth.

Clinical diagnosis of periodontal disease is based on an oral examination, consisting of inspection of the gingival tissue on the buccal and lingual side of every tooth, conducting a periodontal screening and recording pocket depths for each tooth, checking attachment level, measuring plaque index, testing bleeding on probing, testing tooth mobility, and taking radiographs to assess bone loss. Caries are also clinically diagnosed on visual examination and by taking radiographs. In both oral diseases, identification of the etiologic agents may be carried out. For this, oral specimens including plaque, GCF, and saliva are sent to and analyzed in diagnostic laboratories. Isolation of bacterial species from oral specimens using classical in vitro methods is only possible for cultivable species such as *Porphyromonas gingivalis*, *Treponema denticola*, and *Tannerella forsythia* present as a complex biofilm in destructive periodontitis,[131] and *Streptococcus mutans* and *Lactobacillus* sp frequently found in caries.[132,133] However, the majority of the oral bacterial species are uncultivable. For instance, the oral microbiota contains more than 700 individual taxa with approximately 200 characterized bacterial species and only about 100 of them representing cultivable strains in vitro. To bridge this gap, novel approaches in salivary diagnostics have been developed to characterize the role of the uncultivable microbiome in disease initiation and progression. Other studies are conducting a comparative analysis of salivary proteomic profiles in patients with periodontitis and healthy subjects, showing distinctive profiles with alterations of salivary proteins in the presence of periodontal inflammation, which may contribute to the improvement of periodontal diagnosis.[134–136] Recently, a clinical study was conducted in which 100 individuals were enrolled either into a group of healthy/gingivitis subjects or into a group of subjects with periodontitis to identify pathogen and host-response salivary biomarkers correlated with periodontitis.[137] For this purpose, a rapid POC chairside diagnostics was utilized, which had the capacity to characterize early stages of periodontal infection and its progression to disease. Whole saliva was collected and analyzed using antibody arrays to measure the levels of multiple proinflammatory cytokines and bone resorptive/turnover markers. Salivary biomarker data were correlated to comprehensive clinical, radiographic, and microbial plaque biofilm level (measured by quantitative PCR) to generate periodontal disease identification models. As previously described, biomarkers such as MMP-8 and -9 (matrix metalloproteinases) were elevated in subjects with advanced periodontitis, which was predicted when assessing multiple combinations of salivary biomarkers (eg, MMP-8 and -9 and osteoprotegerin) along with red-complex anaerobic periodontal pathogens (eg, *Porphyromonas gingivalis* or *Treponema denticola*). In addition, disease severity was also predicted when obtaining elevated salivary MMP-8 and *T denticola* biofilm levels. This approach proved the usefulness of monitoring salivary and host-response biomarkers for an oral disease. Studies are ongoing to apply this approach to the longitudinal predictions of disease activity.[137] A similar POC diagnostic approach was previously developed as a portable microfluidic device consisting of a chip-based immunoassay to detect biomarkers of periodontal disease in saliva.[138]

The clinical value of salivary proteomic biomarkers in periodontal disease diagnosis is under experimental development and is based on profile changes in molecules involved in inflammation, collagen degradation, and bone loss.[65,137,139] Despite this progress, some of the biomarkers identified are not disease specific. As with salivary proteomics, salivary transcriptomics and genomics in high-throughput platforms have also been developed using oral diseases as models,[65] but face similar challenges as described above.

In addition to using plaque specimens for conventional bacterial isolation methods and saliva samples for proteomic biomarker profiling, GCF specimens have also been tested by ELISA to assess differential expression of specific host biomarkers (eg, RANKL and cathepsin-K indicators of osteoclast activity) for the experimental diagnosis of periodontal disease,[140,141] demonstrating the use of GCF specimens in oral diagnostics. In fact, detection of GCF constituents (mostly inflammatory mediators) in saliva is the current focus of most saliva-based tests for periodontal disease.

The value of salivary diagnostics in caries has also been reported. An experimental assay was developed using biomarkers (genetically determined oligosaccharide profiles present on salivary glycoproteins) for caries risk assessment with prognostic value for caries susceptibility.[142,143] Evaluation of this unique assay is under way for future diagnostic applications.

SUMMARY

Early studies attempting to use saliva as a diagnostic fluid were hampered by a lack of understanding of how these biomarkers enter saliva, the difficulty in detecting some markers owing to low levels in saliva as compared with serum, and lack of attention to the method of collection and storage of samples before analysis. These challenges have largely been met as a result of careful studies of salivary gland physiology, development of sensitive amplification methods (eg, ELISA, qRT-PCR), and education of the scientific community in the methodology for obtaining and dealing with salivary samples. The recent advances in oral fluid biomarker diagnostics have been fueled by novel molecular approaches (eg, proteomics, transcriptomics, and genomics) and metagenomic analyses that have broadened the discovery of microbial pathogens associated with systemic and oral diseases. Similarly, these experimental approaches have been successfully used in the diagnosis of noninfectious systemic and oral conditions (eg, cancers, autoimmune diseases, renal disease, and diabetes). The future of this field will depend on further validation of disease-specific (and stage-specific) biomarkers and their incorporation into state-of-the-art, multiplex assays that are versatile, quantitative, reliable, sensitive, specific, rapid, robust, and cost-effective for broad implementation in diagnostic programs.

ACKNOWLEDGMENTS

The authors acknowledge the contribution of Dr William Abrams in preparing the figures and reviewing the manuscript.

REFERENCES

1. Corstjens PLAM, Malamud D. Point-of-care diagnostics for infectious diseases. In: Wong DT, editor. Saliva diagnostics. Ames (IA): Wiley-Blackwell; 2008. p. 243–54.

2. Farnaud SJ, Kosti O, Getting SJ, et al. Saliva: physiology and diagnostic potential in health and disease. Scientific World Journal 2010;10:434–56.
3. Malamud D, Tabak LA, editors. Saliva as a diagnostic fluid. Ann NY Acad Sci 1993;694.
4. Malamud D, Niedbala RS, New York Academy of Sciences. Oral-based diagnostics. Boston: Blackwell Pub. on behalf of the New York Academy of Sciences; 2007.
5. Wong D. Salivary diagnostics. Ames (IA): Wiley-Blackwell; 2008.
6. Greenberg BL, Glick M, Frantsve-Hawley J, et al. Dentists' attitudes toward chairside screening for medical conditions. J Am Dent Assoc 2010;141(1): 52–62.
7. Parisi MR, Soldini L, Di Perri G, et al. Offer of rapid testing and alternative biological samples as practical tools to implement HIV screening programs. New Microbiol 2009;32(4):391–6.
8. White DA, Scribner AN, Huang JV. A comparison of patient acceptance of fingerstick whole blood and oral fluid rapid HIV screening in an emergency department. J Acquir Immune Defic Syndr 2009;52(1):75–8.
9. Lijnen I, Willems G. DNA research in forensic dentistry. Methods Find Exp Clin Pharmacol 2001;23(9):511–7.
10. Virkler K, Lednev IK. Analysis of body fluids for forensic purposes: from laboratory testing to non-destructive rapid confirmatory identification at a crime scene. Forensic Sci Int 2009;188(1–3):1–17.
11. Kohnemann S, Pfeiffer H. Application of mtDNA SNP analysis in forensic casework. Forensic Sci Int Genet 2010. [Epub ahead of print].
12. Gerritsen L, Geerlings MI, Beekman AT, et al. Early and late life events and salivary cortisol in older persons. Psychol Med 2010;40(9):1569–78.
13. Hedriana HL, Munro CJ, Eby-Wilkens EM, et al. Changes in rates of salivary estriol increases before parturition at term. Am J Obstet Gynecol 2001;184(2): 123–30.
14. Kim MS, Lee YJ, Ahn RS. Day-to-day differences in cortisol levels and molar cortisol-to-DHEA ratios among working individuals. Yonsei Med J 2010;51(2): 212–8.
15. Klebanoff MA, Meis PJ, Dombrowski MP, et al. Salivary progesterone and estriol among pregnant women treated with 17-alpha-hydroxyprogesterone caproate or placebo. Am J Obstet Gynecol 2008;199(5):506, e501–7.
16. Matchock RL, Dorn LD, Susman EJ. Diurnal and seasonal cortisol, testosterone, and DHEA rhythms in boys and girls during puberty. Chronobiol Int 2007;24(5): 969–90.
17. Touitou Y, Auzeby A, Camus F, et al. Daily profiles of salivary and urinary melatonin and steroids in healthy prepubertal boys. J Pediatr Endocrinol Metab 2009;22(11):1009–15.
18. Abrams WR, Barber CA, McCann K, et al. Development of a microfluidic device for detection of pathogens in oral samples using upconverting phosphor technology (UPT). Ann N Y Acad Sci 2007;1098:375–88.
19. Groschl M. The physiological role of hormones in saliva. BioEssays 2009;31: 843–52.
20. Gau V, Wong D. Oral fluid nanosensor test (OFNASET) with advanced electrochemical-based molecular analysis platform. Ann N Y Acad Sci 2007;1098: 401–10.
21. Walt DR, Blicharz TM, Hayman RB, et al. Microsensor arrays for saliva diagnostics. Ann N Y Acad Sci 2007;1098:389–400.

22. Brandtzaeg P. Do salivary antibodies reliably reflect both mucosal and systemic immunity? Ann N Y Acad Sci 2007;1098:288–311.
23. Dias Fernandes CS, Salum FG, Bandeira D, et al. Salivary dehydroepiandrosterone (DHEA) levels in patients with the complaint of burning mouth: a case-control study. Oral Surg Oral Med Oral Pathol Oral Radiol Endod 2009;108(4):537–43.
24. Gavrilova N, Lindau ST. Salivary sex hormone measurement in a national, population-based study of older adults. J Gerontol B Psychol Sci Soc Sci 2009;64(Suppl 1):i94–105.
25. Gray SH, Ebe LK, Feldman HA, et al. Salivary progesterone levels before menarche: a prospective study of adolescent girls. J Clin Endocrinol Metab 2010;95:3507–11.
26. Hamilton LD, van Anders SM, Cox DN, et al. The effect of competition on salivary testosterone in elite female athletes. Int J Sports Physiol Perform 2009; 4(4):538–42.
27. Manolopoulou J, Gerum S, Mulatero P, et al. Salivary aldosterone as a diagnostic aid in primary aldosteronism. Horm Metab Res 2010;42:400–5.
28. Vitzthum VJ, Worthman CM, Beall CM, et al. Seasonal and circadian variation in salivary testosterone in rural Bolivian men. Am J Human Biol 2009;21(6):762–8.
29. Warrener L, Slibinskas R, Brown D, et al. Development and evaluation of a rapid immunochromatographic test for mumps-specific IgM in oral fluid specimens and use as a matrix for preserving viral nucleic acid for RT-PCR. J Med Virol 2010;82(3):485–93.
30. Adisen E, Aral A, Aybay C, et al. Salivary epidermal growth factor levels in Behcet's disease and recurrent aphthous stomatitis. Dermatology 2008;217(3): 235–40.
31. Eckley CA, Rios Lda S, Rizzo LV. Salivary EGF concentration in adults with reflux chronic laryngitis before and after treatment: preliminary results. Braz J Otorhinolaryngol 2007;73(2):156–60.
32. Nam JW, Chung JW, Kho HS, et al. Nerve growth factor concentration in human saliva. Oral Dis 2007;13(2):187–92.
33. Taichman NS, Cruchley AT, Fletcher LM, et al. Vascular endothelial growth factor in normal human salivary glands and saliva: a possible role in the maintenance of mucosal homeostasis. Lab Invest 1998;78(7):869–75.
34. Upile T, Jerjes W, Kafas P, et al. Salivary VEGF: a non-invasive angiogenic and lymphangiogenic proxy in head and neck cancer prognostication. Int Arch Med 2009;2(1):12.
35. Blicharz TM, Rissin DM, Bowden M, et al. Use of colorimetric test strips for monitoring the effect of hemodialysis on salivary nitrite and uric acid in patients with end-stage renal disease: a proof of principle. Clin Chem 2008;54(9):1473–80.
36. Suh KI, Kim YK, Kho HS. Salivary levels of IL-1beta, IL-6, IL-8, and TNF-alpha in patients with burning mouth syndrome. Arch Oral Biol 2009;54(9):797–802.
37. Teles RP, Likhari V, Socransky SS, et al. Salivary cytokine levels in subjects with chronic periodontitis and in periodontally healthy individuals: a cross-sectional study. J Periodont Res 2009;44(3):411–7.
38. Thomas MV, Branscum A, Miller CS, et al. Within-subject variability in repeated measures of salivary analytes in healthy adults. J Periodontol 2009;80(7): 1146–53.
39. Roescher N, Tak PP, Illei GG. Cytokines in Sjogren's syndrome. Oral Dis 2009; 15(8):519–26.
40. Malamud D, Abrams WR, Bau H, et al. Oral-based techniques for the diagnosis of infectious diseases. J Calif Dent Assoc 2006;34(4):297–301.

41. Palanisamy V, Sharma S, Deshpande A, et al. Nanostructural and transcriptomic analyses of human saliva derived exosomes. PLoS One 2010;5(1):e8577.

42. Starke EM, Smoot JC, Wu JH, et al. Saliva-based diagnostics using 16S rRNA microarrays and microfluidics. Ann N Y Acad Sci 2007;1098:345–61.

43. Zimmermann BG, Park NJ, Wong DT. Genomic targets in saliva. Ann N Y Acad Sci 2007;1098:184–91.

44. Qvarnstrom M, Janket S, Jones JA, et al. Salivary lysozyme and prevalent hypertension. J Dent Res 2008;87(5):480–4.

45. Yan W, Apweiler R, Balgley BM, et al. Systematic comparison of the human saliva and plasma proteomes. Proteomics Clin Appl 2009;3(1):116–34.

46. Zehetbauer S, Wojahn T, Hiller KA, et al. Resemblance of salivary protein profiles between children with early childhood caries and caries-free controls. Eur J Oral Sci 2009;117(4):369–73.

47. Bosker WM, Huestis MA. Oral fluid testing for drugs of abuse. Clin Chem 2009; 55(11):1910–31.

48. Drummer OH. Drug testing in oral fluid. Clin Biochem Rev 2006;27(3):147–59.

49. Langel K, Engblom C, Pehrsson A, et al. Drug testing in oral fluid-evaluation of sample collection devices. J Anal Toxicol 2008;32(6):393–401.

50. Langman LJ. The use of oral fluid for therapeutic drug management: clinical and forensic toxicology. Ann N Y Acad Sci 2007;1098:145–66.

51. Floriano PN, Christodoulides N, Miller CS, et al. Use of saliva-based nano-biochip tests for acute myocardial infarction at the point of care: a feasibility study. Clin Chem 2009;55(8):1530–8.

52. Meurman JH. Infectious and dietary risk factors of oral cancer. Oral Oncol 2010; 46:411–3.

53. Miller CS, Foley JD, Bailey AL, et al. Current developments in salivary diagnostics. Biomark Med 2010;4(1):171–89.

54. Arregger AL, Cardoso EM, Tumilasci O, et al. Diagnostic value of salivary cortisol in end stage renal disease. Steroids 2008;73(1):77–82.

55. Nagler RM. Saliva analysis for monitoring dialysis and renal function. Clin Chem 2008;54(9):1415–7.

56. Savica V, Calo L, Santoro D, et al. Salivary phosphate secretion in chronic kidney disease. J Ren Nutr 2008;18(1):87–90.

57. Savica V, Calo LA, Granata A, et al. A new approach to the evaluation of hyperphosphatemia in chronic kidney disease. Clin Nephrol 2007;68(4):216–21.

58. Dabbs JM Jr. Salivary testosterone measurements in behavioral studies. Ann N Y Acad Sci 1993;694:177–83.

59. Azuma M, Kasai Y, Tamatani T, et al. Involvement of p53 mutation in the development of human salivary gland pleomorphic adenomas. Cancer Lett 1992; 65(1):61–71.

60. Streckfus C, Bigler L, Tucci M, et al. A preliminary study of CA15-3, c-erbB-2, epidermal growth factor receptor, cathepsin-D, and p53 in saliva among women with breast carcinoma. Cancer Invest 2000;18(2):101–9.

61. Streckfus C, Bigler L. The use of soluble, salivary c-erbB-2 for the detection and post-operative follow-up of breast cancer in women: the results of a five-year translational research study. Adv Dent Res 2005;18(1):17–24.

62. Chen DX, Schwartz PE, Li FQ. Saliva and serum CA 125 assays for detecting malignant ovarian tumors. Obstet Gynecol 1990;75(4):701–4.

63. Blackburn AC, Hill LZ, Roberts AL, et al. Genetic mapping in mice identifies DMBT1 as a candidate modifier of mammary tumors and breast cancer risk. Am J Pathol 2007;170(6):2030–41.

64. Braidotti P, Nuciforo PG, Mollenhauer J, et al. DMBT1 expression is down-regulated in breast cancer. BMC Cancer 2004;4:46.
65. Zhang L, Henson BS, Camargo PM, et al. The clinical value of salivary biomarkers for periodontal disease. Periodontol 2000, 2009;51:25–37.
66. Rao PV, Reddy AP, Lu X, et al. Proteomic identification of salivary biomarkers of type-2 diabetes. J Proteome Res 2009;8(1):239–45.
67. Novak BJ, Blake DR, Meinardi S, et al. Exhaled methyl nitrate as a noninvasive marker of hyperglycemia in type 1 diabetes. Proc Natl Acad Sci U S A 2007; 104(40):15613–8.
68. Strauss SM, Wheeler AJ, Russell SL, et al. The potential use of gingival crevicular blood for measuring glucose to screen for diabetes: an examination based on characteristics of the blood collection site. J Periodontol 2009;80(6):907–14.
69. Whitcher JP, Shiboski CH, Shiboski SC, et al. A simplified quantitative method for assessing keratoconjunctivitis sicca from the Sjogren's Syndrome International Registry. Am J Ophthalmol 2010;149(3):405–15.
70. Pillemer SR, Matteson EL, Jacobsson LT, et al. Incidence of physician-diagnosed primary Sjogren's syndrome in residents of Olmsted County, Minnesota. Mayo Clin Proc 2001;76(6):593–9.
71. Cummins MJ, Papas A, Kammer GM, et al. Treatment of primary Sjogren's syndrome with low-dose human interferon alfa administered by the oromucosal route: combined phase III results. Arthritis Rheum 2003;49(4):585–93.
72. Kruszka P, O'Brian RJ. Diagnosis and management of Sjogren's syndrome. Am Fam Physician 2009;79(6):465–70.
73. Hu S, Wang J, Meijer J, et al. Salivary proteomic and genomic biomarkers for primary Sjogren's syndrome. Arthritis Rheum 2007;56(11):3588–600.
74. Denny P, Hagen FK, Hardt M, et al. The proteomes of human parotid and submandibular/sublingual gland salivas collected as the ductal secretions. J Proteome Res 2008;7(5):1994–2006.
75. Hu S, Xie Y, Ramachandran P, et al. Large-scale identification of proteins in human salivary proteome by liquid chromatography/mass spectrometry and two-dimensional gel electrophoresis-mass spectrometry. Proteomics 2005;5(6):1714–28.
76. Sondej M, Denny PA, Xie Y, et al. Glycoprofiling of the human salivary proteome. Clin Proteomics 2009;5(1):52–68.
77. Zheng M, Li L, Tang YL, et al. Biomarkers in tongue cancer: understanding the molecular basis and their clinical implications. Postgrad Med J 2010;86(1015):292–8.
78. Petersen PE. Oral cancer prevention and control—the approach of the World Health Organization. Oral Oncol 2009;45(4–5):454–60.
79. Tshering Vogel DW, Zbaeren P, Thoeny HC. Cancer of the oral cavity and oropharynx. Cancer Imaging 2010;10:62–72.
80. Guneri P, Epstein JB, Ergun S, et al. Toluidine blue color perception in identification of oral mucosal lesions. Clin Oral Investig 2010. [Epub ahead of print].
81. Seoane Leston J, Diz Dios P. Diagnostic clinical aids in oral cancer. Oral Oncol 2010;46:418–22.
82. Xie H, Onsongo G, Popko J, et al. Proteomics analysis of cells in whole saliva from oral cancer patients via value-added three-dimensional peptide fractionation and tandem mass spectrometry. Mol Cell Proteomics 2008;7(3):486–98.
83. Williams MD. Integration of biomarkers including molecular targeted therapies in head and neck cancer. Head Neck Pathol 2010;4(1):62–9.
84. Sugimoto M, Wong DT, Hirayama A, et al. Capillary electrophoresis mass spectrometry-based saliva metabolomics identified oral, breast and pancreatic cancer-specific profiles. Metabolomics 2010;6(1):78–95.

85. Lee JM, Garon E, Wong DT. Salivary diagnostics. Orthod Craniofac Res 2009; 12(3):206–11.
86. Hu S, Arellano M, Boontheung P, et al. Salivary proteomics for oral cancer biomarker discovery. Clin Cancer Res 2008;14(19):6246–52.
87. Bigler LR, Streckfus CF, Dubinsky WP. Salivary biomarkers for the detection of malignant tumors that are remote from the oral cavity. Clin Lab Med 2009; 29(1):71–85.
88. Bilodeau E, Alawi F, Costello BJ, et al. Molecular diagnostics for head and neck pathology. Oral Maxillofac Surg Clin North Am 2010;22(1):183–94.
89. Ghannoum MA, Jurevic RJ, Mukherjee PK, et al. Characterization of the oral fungal microbiome (mycobiome) in healthy individuals. PLoS Pathog 2010; 6(1):e1000713.
90. Samaranayake LP, Keung Leung W, Jin L. Oral mucosal fungal infections. Periodontol 2000, 2009;49:39–59.
91. Richardson R, Antilla VJ. [Diagnosis and treatment of oral candidosis]. Duodecim 2010;126(2):174–80 [in Finnish].
92. Iatta R, Napoli C, Borghi E, et al. Rare mycoses of the oral cavity: a literature epidemiologic review. Oral Surg Oral Med Oral Pathol Oral Radiol Endod 2009;108(5):647–55.
93. Terai H, Shimahara M. Usefulness of culture test and direct examination for the diagnosis of oral atrophic candidiasis. Int J Dermatol 2009;48(4):371–3.
94. Kurita H, Kamata T, Zhao C, et al. Usefulness of a commercial enzyme-linked immunosorbent assay kit for Candida mannan antigen for detecting Candida in oral rinse solutions. Oral Surg Oral Med Oral Pathol Oral Radiol Endod 2009;107(4):531–4.
95. Naglik JR, Scott J, Rahman D, et al. Serum and saliva antibodies do not inhibit *Candida albicans* Sap2 proteinase activity using a BSA hydrolysis assay. Med Mycol 2005;43(1):73–7.
96. Pomarico L, Cerqueira DF, de Araujo Soares RM, et al. Associations among the use of highly active antiretroviral therapy, oral candidiasis, oral *Candida* species and salivary immunoglobulin A in HIV-infected children. Oral Surg Oral Med Oral Pathol Oral Radiol Endod 2009;108(2):203–10.
97. Pomarico L, de Souza IP, Castro GF, et al. Levels of salivary IgA antibodies to *Candida* spp. in HIV-infected adult patients: a systematic review. J Dent 2010; 38(1):10–5.
98. Andrews E, Seaman WT, Webster-Cyriaque J. Oropharyngeal carcinoma in nonsmokers and non-drinkers: a role for HPV. Oral Oncol 2009;45(6):486–91.
99. Andrews E, Shores C, Hayes DN, et al. Concurrent human papillomavirus-associated tonsillar carcinoma in 2 couples. J Infect Dis 2009;200(6):882–7.
100. Gennaro S, Naidoo S, Berthold P. Oral health & HIV/AIDS. MCN Am J Matern Child Nurs 2008;33(1):50–7.
101. Grande SR, Imbronito AV, Okuda OS, et al. Herpes viruses in periodontal compromised sites: comparison between HIV-positive and -negative patients. J Clin Periodontol 2008;35(10):838–45.
102. Heinic GS, Greenspan D, Greenspan JS. Oral CMV lesions and the HIV infected. Early recognition can help prevent morbidity. J Am Dent Assoc 1993; 124(2):99–105.
103. Hille JJ, Webster-Cyriaque J, Palefski JM, et al. Mechanisms of expression of HHV8, EBV and HPV in selected HIV-associated oral lesions. Oral Dis 2002; 8(Suppl 2):161–8.
104. Itin PH, Lautenschlager S. Viral lesions of the mouth in HIV-infected patients. Dermatology 1997;194(1):1–7.

105. Merchant VA. An update on the herpesviruses. J Calif Dent Assoc 1996;24(1): 38–46.
106. Reichart PA. Oral ulcerations in HIV infection. Oral Dis 1997;3(Suppl 1):S180–2.
107. Ramirez-Amador VA, Espinosa E, Gonzalez-Ramirez I, et al. Identification of oral candidosis, hairy leukoplakia and recurrent oral ulcers as distinct cases of immune reconstitution inflammatory syndrome. Int J STD AIDS 2009;20(4):259–61.
108. Shiboski CH, Patton LL, Webster-Cyriaque JY, et al. The Oral HIV/AIDS research alliance: updated case definitions of oral disease endpoints. J Oral Pathol Med 2009;38(6):481–8.
109. Chen D, Mauk M, Qiu X, et al. An integrated, self-contained microfluidic cassette for isolation, amplification, and detection of nucleic acids. Biomed Microdevices 2010;12(4):705–19.
110. Chohan BH, Lavreys L, Mandaliya KN, et al. Validation of a modified commercial enzyme-linked immunoassay for detection of human immunodeficiency virus type 1 immunoglobulin G antibodies in saliva. Clin Diagn Lab Immunol 2001; 8(2):346–8.
111. Liu C, Qiu X, Ongagna S, et al. A timer-actuated immunoassay cassette for detecting molecular markers in oral fluids. Lab Chip 2009;9(6):768–76.
112. Qiu X, Thompson JA, Chen Z, et al. Finger-actuated, self-contained immunoassay cassettes. Biomed Microdevices 2009;11(6):1175–86.
113. Sherman GG, Lilian RR, Coovadia AH. Oral fluid tests for screening of human immunodeficiency virus-exposed infants. Pediatr Infect Dis J 2010;29(2):169–72.
114. Whitney JB, Luedemann C, Bao S, et al. Monitoring HIV vaccine trial participants for primary infection: studies in the SIV/macaque model. AIDS 2009;23(12): 1453–60.
115. Wu X, Jackson S. Plasma and salivary IgA subclasses and IgM in HIV-1-infected individuals. J Clin Immunol 2002;22(2):106–15.
116. Yapijakis C, Panis V, Koufaliotis N, et al. Immunological and molecular detection of human immunodeficiency virus in saliva, and comparison with blood testing. Eur J Oral Sci 2006;114(3):175–9.
117. Gardner MS, Rowland MD, Siu AY, et al. Comprehensive defensin assay for saliva. Anal Chem 2009;81(2):557–66.
118. Adamopoulou M, Vairaktaris E, Panis V, et al. HPV detection rate in saliva may depend on the immune system efficiency. In Vivo 2008;22(5):599–602.
119. Chuang AY, Chuang TC, Chang S, et al. Presence of HPV DNA in convalescent salivary rinses is an adverse prognostic marker in head and neck squamous cell carcinoma. Oral Oncol 2008;44(10):915–9.
120. Cameron JE, Snowhite IV, Chaturvedi AK, et al. Human papillomavirus-specific antibody status in oral fluids modestly reflects serum status in human immunodeficiency virus-positive individuals. Clin Diagn Lab Immunol 2003;10(3):431–8.
121. Idesawa M, Sugano N, Ikeda K, et al. Detection of Epstein-Barr virus in saliva by real-time PCR. Oral Microbiol Immunol 2004;19(4):230–2.
122. Ling PD, Vilchez RA, Keitel WA, et al. Epstein-Barr virus DNA loads in adult human immunodeficiency virus type 1-infected patients receiving highly active antiretroviral therapy. Clin Infect Dis 2003;37(9):1244–9.
123. Mbulaiteye SM, Walters M, Engels EA, et al. High levels of Epstein-Barr virus DNA in saliva and peripheral blood from Ugandan mother-child pairs. J Infect Dis 2006;193(3):422–6.
124. Imbronito AV, Grande SR, Freitas NM, et al. Detection of Epstein-Barr virus and human cytomegalovirus in blood and oral samples: comparison of three sampling methods. J Oral Sci 2008;50(1):25–31.

125. Yamamoto AY, Mussi-Pinhata MM, Marin LJ, et al. Is saliva as reliable as urine for detection of cytomegalovirus DNA for neonatal screening of congenital CMV infection? J Clin Virol 2006;36(3):228–30.

126. Grosjean J, Hantz S, Cotin S, et al. Direct genotyping of cytomegalovirus envelope glycoproteins from toddler's saliva samples. J Clin Virol 2009;46(Suppl 4): S43–8.

127. Raggam RB, Wagner J, Michelin BD, et al. Reliable detection and quantitation of viral nucleic acids in oral fluid: Liquid phase-based sample collection in conjunction with automated and standardized molecular assays. J Med Virol 2008;80(9):1684–8.

128. Gandhi M, Koelle DM, Ameli N, et al. Prevalence of human herpesvirus-8 salivary shedding in HIV increases with CD4 count. J Dent Res 2004;83(8):639–43.

129. Widmer IC, Erb P, Grob H, et al. Human herpesvirus 8 oral shedding in HIV-infected men with and without Kaposi sarcoma. J Acquir Immune Defic Syndr 2006;42(4):420–5.

130. Mancuso R, Biffi R, Valli M, et al. HHV8 a subtype is associated with rapidly evolving classic Kaposi's sarcoma. J Med Virol 2008;80(12):2153–60.

131. Holt SC, Ebersole JL. *Porphyromonas gingivalis, Treponema denticola*, and *Tannerella forsythia*: the "red complex", a prototype polybacterial pathogenic consortium in periodontitis. Periodontol 2000, 2005;38:72–122.

132. Kanasi E, Johansson I, Lu SC, et al. Microbial risk markers for childhood caries in pediatricians' offices. J Dent Res 2010;89(4):378–83.

133. Wen ZT, Yates D, Ahn SJ, et al. Biofilm formation and virulence expression by Streptococcus mutans are altered when grown in dual-species model. BMC Microbiol 2010;10:111.

134. Goncalves Lda R, Soares MR, Nogueira FC, et al. Comparative proteomic analysis of whole saliva from chronic periodontitis patients. J Proteomics 2010;73(7): 1334–41.

135. Haigh BJ, Stewart KW, Whelan JR, et al. Alterations in the salivary proteome associated with periodontitis. J Clin Periodontol 2010;37(3):241–7.

136. Wu Y, Shu R, Luo LJ, et al. Initial comparison of proteomic profiles of whole unstimulated saliva obtained from generalized aggressive periodontitis patients and healthy control subjects. J Periodont Res 2009;44(5):636–44.

137. Ramseier CA, Kinney JS, Herr AE, et al. Identification of pathogen and host-response markers correlated with periodontal disease. J Periodontol 2009; 80(3):436–46.

138. Herr AE, Hatch AV, Giannobile WV, et al. Integrated microfluidic platform for oral diagnostics. Ann N Y Acad Sci 2007;1098:362–74.

139. Koss MA, Castro CE, Salum KM, et al. Changes in saliva protein composition in patients with periodontal disease. Acta Odontol Latinoam 2009;22(2):105–12.

140. Mogi M, Otogoto J. Expression of cathepsin-K in gingival crevicular fluid of patients with periodontitis. Arch Oral Biol 2007;52(9):894–8.

141. Mogi M, Otogoto J, Ota N, et al. Differential expression of RANKL and osteoprotegerin in gingival crevicular fluid of patients with periodontitis. J Dent Res 2004; 83(2):166–9.

142. Denny PC. A saliva-based prognostic test for dental caries susceptibility. J Dent Hyg 2009;83(4):175–6.

143. Denny PC, Denny PA, Takashima J, et al. A novel saliva test for caries risk assessment. J Calif Dent Assoc 2006;34(4):287–90, 292–4.

Index

Note: Page numbers of article titles are in **boldface** type.

Dent Clin N Am 55 (2011) 179–185
doi:10.1016/S0011-8532(10)00115-1
0011-8532/11/$ – see front matter © 2011 Elsevier Inc. All rights reserved.

dental.theclinics.com

Printed and bound by CPI Group (UK) Ltd, Croydon, CR0 4YY

03/10/2024

01040459-0017